KETO DIET WOMEN OVER 50

THE COMPLETE GUIDE + EASY AND DELICIOUS RECIPES TO EMBRACE THE KETO LIFESTYLE, LIVE HEALTHIER WITH MORE ENERGY

Gracelynn Rogers

Table of Contents

Chapter 4

WHAT FOODS TO AVOID IN THE KETO DIET AND WHY?

Chapter 5

DOES KETO DIET HAVE SIDE EFFECTS?

Keto Breath

Keto Flu

Fatigue

GI Side Effects

Weakened Immune System

Vitamin and Other Mineral Deficiencies

Increased Risk of Chronic Disease

Chronic Inflammation

The Challenge of Weight Cycling

Chapter 6

BREAKFAST RECIPES

Yogurt Waffles

Broccoli Muffins

Pumpkin Bread

Spinach Artichoke Breakfast Bake

Granola Bars

Chapter 7

LUNCH RECIPES

Mushroom & Cauliflower Risotto

Chapter 8

DINNER RECIPES

CHOCOLATE CHIA PUDDING

KETO MUFFINS

BLUEBERRY WAFFLES

KETO PANCAKES

JALAPENO POPPER EGG CUPS

SAVORY CHEDDAR OMELET

SPINACH & FETA BREAKFAST WRAPS

AVOCADO TOASTS WITH 3 TOPPINGS

SOUP & STEW RECIPES

EASY SUMMER GAZPACHO

FRESH AVOCADO SOUP

COLD ITALIAN CUCUMBER SOUP

TOMATO SOUP & GRILLED CHEESE SANDWICHES

CREAMY TAHINI ZOODLE SOUP

GREEK EGG LEMON CHICKEN SOUP

CAULIFLOWER RICE & CHICKEN SOUP

ASPARAGUS PUREE SOUP

CREAMY CHICKEN POT PIE SOUP

CHUNKY PORK SOUP

CABBAGE SOUP WITH BEEF

MAIN RECIPES

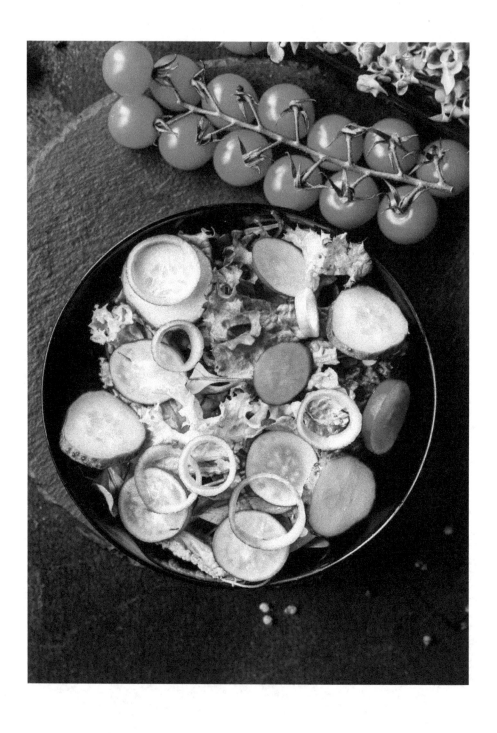

Introduction

What is a Keto Diet?

The name "Keto" comes from the word "ketogenic" which refers to the metabolic state of ketosis that starts in the body when carbohydrate intake is suddenly reduced and replaced with healthy fats. Most people start a ketogenic diet to lose weight, not just in water weight but in abdominal and other stored fat. It resembles the Atkins and other low-carb diets. The primary guideline is to drastically reduce your consumption of carbohydrates and replace them with healthy fats. This dramatic reduction in carbohydrates helps your body enter a metabolic state called ketosis in which your body burns fat for fuel rather than glucose.

The average person eats foods loaded in carbohydrates; the liver then converts glucose. Your body creates insulin in order to move the glucose into the bloodstream, which distributes it throughout your body and brain. The body's primary source of energy is glucose whenever carbohydrates are present in the body. Your body will always use glucose over fat or any other energy source.

The keto diet is focused on not using glucose as your energy source but instead fat. Once your body enters ketosis, your body becomes effective at burning fat, losing weight, and overall improving health. It also converts fat into ketones inside your liver, which can supply energy for the brain. The ketogenic diet can cause also cause a massive reduction in blood sugar and insulin levels.

The keto diet or the ketogenic diet requires you to follow a meal plan that is low in carbs and high in fat. It has some similarities with diet plans like the Atkin's diet and other low-carb meal plans. The goal of this diet is to increase the fat content in the body and reducing the carbohydrate content to push your body into the ketosis state which turns you into a fat burning machine.

Part 1

Chapter 1

BENEFITS OF KETO DIET FOR WOMEN OVER 50

The Keto diet has become so popular in recent years because of the success people have noticed. Not only have they lost weight, but scientific studies show that the Keto diet can help you improve your health in many others. As when starting any new diet or exercise routine, there may seem to be some disadvantages, so we will go over those for the Keto diet. But most people agree that the benefits outweigh the change period!

Benefits/Advantages

Losing Weight

For most people, this is the foremost benefit of switching to Keto! Their previous diet method may have stalled for them, or they were noticing weight creeping back on. With Keto, studies have shown that people have been able to follow this diet and relay fewer hunger pangs and suppressed appetite while losing weight at the same time! You are minimizing your carbohydrate intake, which means more occasional blood sugar spikes. Often, those fluctuations in blood sugar levels make you feel hungrier and more prone to snacking in between meals. Instead, by guiding the body towards ketosis, you are eating a more fulfilling diet of fat and protein and harnessing energy from ketone molecules instead of glucose. Studies show that low-carb diets effectively reduce visceral fat (the fat you commonly see around the abdomen increases as you become obese). This reduces your risk of obesity and improves your health in the long run.

Reduce the Risk of Type 2 Diabetes

The problem with carbohydrates is how unstable they make blood sugar levels. This can be very dangerous for people who have diabetes or are pre-diabetic because of unbalanced blood sugar levels or family history. Keto is an excellent option because of the minimal intake of carbohydrates it requires. Instead, you are harnessing most of your calories from fat or protein, which will not cause blood sugar spikes and, ultimately, less pressured the pancreas to secrete insulin. Many studies have found that diabetes patients who followed the Keto diet lost more weight and eventually reduced their fasting glucose levels. This is monumental news for patients with unstable blood sugar levels or hopes to avoid or reduce their diabetes medication intake.

Improve Cardiovascular Risk Symptoms to Lower Your Chances of Having Heart Disease

Most people assume that following Keto that is so high in fat content has to increase your risk of coronary heart disease or heart attack. But the research proves otherwise! Research shows that switching to Keto can lower your blood pressure, increase your HDL good cholesterol, and reduce your triglyceride fatty acid levels. That's because the fat you are consuming on Keto is healthy and high-quality fats, so they reverse many unhealthy symptoms of heart disease. They boost your "good" HDL cholesterol numbers and decrease your "bad" LDL cholesterol numbers. It also reduces the level of triglyceride fatty acids in the bloodstream. A top-level of these can lead to stroke, heart attack, or premature death. And what are the top levels of fatty acids linked to?

High Consumption of Carbohydrates

With the Keto diet, you are drastically cutting your intake of carbohydrates to improve fatty acid levels and improve other risk factors. A 2018 study on the Keto diet found that it can improve 22 out of 26 risk factors for cardiovascular heart disease! These factors can be critical to some people, especially those who have a history of heart disease in their family.

Increases the Body's Energy Levels

Let's briefly compare the difference between the glucose molecules synthesized from a high carbohydrate intake versus ketones produced on the Keto diet. The liver makes ketones and use fat molecules you already stored. This makes them much more energy-rich and an endless source of fuel compared to glucose, a simple sugar molecule. These ketones can give you a burst of energy physically and mentally, allowing you to have greater focus, clarity, and attention to detail.

Decreases Inflammation in the Body

Inflammation on its own is a natural response by the body's immune system, but when it becomes uncontrollable, it can lead to an array of health problems, some severe and some minor. The health concerns include acne, autoimmune conditions, arthritis, psoriasis, irritable bowel syndrome, and even acne and eczema. Often, removing sugars and carbohydrates from your diet can help patients of these diseases avoid flare-ups - and the delightful news is Keto does just that! A 2008 research study found that Keto decreased a blood marker linked to high inflammation in the body by nearly 40%. This is glorious news for people who may suffer from inflammatory disease and want to change their diet to improve.

Increases Your Mental Functioning Level

As we elaborated earlier, the energy-rich ketones can boost the body's physical and mental levels of alertness. Research has shown that Keto is a much better energy source for the brain than simple sugar glucose molecules are. With nearly 75% of your diet coming from healthy fats, the brain's neural cells and mitochondria have a better source of energy to function at the highest level. Some studies have tested patients on the Keto diet and found they had higher cognitive functioning, better memory recall, and were less susceptible to memory loss. The Keto diet can even decrease the occurrence of migraines, which can be very detrimental to patients.

Decreases Risk of Diseases like Alzheimer's, Parkinson's, and Epilepsy

They created the Keto diet in the 1920s to combat epilepsy in children. From there, research has found that Keto can improve your cognitive functioning level and protect brain cells from injury or damage. This is very good to reduce the risk of neurodegenerative disease, which begins in the brain because of neural cells mutating and functioning with damaged parts or lower than peak optimal functioning. Studies have found that the following Keto can improve the mental functioning of patients who suffer from diseases like Alzheimer's or Parkinson's. These neurodegenerative diseases sadly have no cure, but the Keto diet could improve symptoms as they progress. Researchers believe that it's because cutting out carbs from your diet, which reduces the occurrence of blood sugar spikes that the body's neural cells have to keep adjusting to.

Keto Can Regulate Hormones in Women Who Have PCOS (Polycystic Ovary Syndrome) and PMS (Pre-Menstrual Syndrome)

Women who have PCOS suffer from infertility, which can be very heartbreaking for young couples trying to start a family. For this condition, there is no known cure, but we believe it's related to many similar diabetic symptoms like obesity and a high level of insulin. This causes the body to produce more sex hormones, which can lead to infertility. The Keto diet paved its way as a popular way to regulate insulin and hormone levels and increase a woman's chances of getting pregnant.

Chapter 2

IMPORTANCE OF LIFESTYLE

Enhance Your Physical Activity

Taking part in physical activity may support ketone fixations during carb restriction. This effect can be improved by working in a quick paced state.

Exercising offers a plethora of benefits to all, regardless of your age! Healthy movement results in improved flexibility and more robust bones, which is quite essential for older folks. You see, as you age, your body's muscle mass starts to decrease. As we enter our fifties, adults begin to lose three to five percent of muscle mass as they enter each new decade.

However, we do realize how the thought of exercising regularly at an older age can seem like a challenge, especially if you're feeling let down with frequent aches and pains. But in many ways, the benefits of exercising outweigh the potential risks. Let's dive into why exercising is such important for seniors.

While you may be having thoughts about exercising, here are a couple of services that you can't ignore:

Prevents Diseases

Regular physical activity has been known to reduce the risks of diseases such as diabetes and heart disease. Mainly because exercise strengthens overall immune functioning, which is particularly beneficial for seniors who are often immunocompromised. Even if you can't hit the gym, some form of light exercise can play an integral role in disease management.

Helps Increase Social Ties and Prevents Isolation

Aging can be a daunting process, but it becomes fun when a community surrounds you. Opting for yoga or fitness classes not only makes exercising more fun, but it also helps you strengthen social ties with other older adults in your neighborhood. It can help ward off the occasional loneliness that one is likely to feel at old age. Plus, this will help you stay committed to your goals and lead a healthier lifestyle.

Improves Cognitive Function

Regular exercise can also improve fine motor skills that boost cognitive function. Several studies have shown how exercising can reduce the risk of dementia.

Tips & Tricks Exercises for Seniors

Here is a list of tips exercises that people in their fifties and beyond can enjoy:

Light Weight Training

You can start with a little weight training to retain bone density and build muscle mass. If you're more interested in doing home exercises than joining the gym, invest in 2-pound weights, perform arm raises, and shoulder presses.

Ideally, we recommend that you join a fitness center or gym where you can meet like-minded folks. You can also get yourself a personal trainer who can guide customized workouts for you. Either way, remember to take it slow at first as you don't want to exert yourself too much.

Walking

If lifting weights isn't for you, good old-fashioned walking should also work for you. Consider taking a nice walk around your neighborhood or go to a park nearby. You'll be able to make some friends and enjoy the weather while you're at it too.

In case you'd rather workout at home, strap on a pedometer, and get going around the house. You'll get more out of this workout if you move your arms and lift your knees as you take each step.

Aerobics

Joining an aerobics class can significantly help you keep your muscles healthy while maintaining mobility. It will not only improve balance but will reduce the risk of falls, thus drastically improving the overall quality of your life as you grow older.

Many studies have also indicated how aerobic exercises can protect memory and sharpen your mind and improving cognitive function among older adults. If you're not comfortable joining a class, you'll find plenty of videos online. Aerobic exercises have also been known to get the heart pumping, improving cardiovascular help.

Swimming

Do you find regular exercise too dull? Swimming is a fun, impact-free exercise that can get yours through the day. It's almost pain-free and won't trouble your aging joints. Swimming offers resistance training and will help you get back up to your feet again.

Here's how it works: the water offers gentle resistance while giving you a cardiovascular workout too. It also builds muscle capacity and helps you build strength again.

Yoga

What's no to love about yoga? It's relaxing, it's healthy, and you can enjoy it with a group. Yoga does an excellent job of improving flexibility in your joints. It allows seniors to remain limber and maintain their sense of balance. If you have trouble moving about or stretching, then you can try chair yoga.

Some classic yoga poses that you might want to try out include seated forward bend, downward facing dog, and warrior.

Squats

When you're working on an exercise program, you shouldn't skip the idea of strength training. Squats happen to be an excellent way to strengthen the muscles of your lower body. Doing squats is relatively easy, and you won't need any sort of equipment except for maybe a chair to support yourself. However, if you have trouble with balance, we suggest you skip this exercise and opt for something much more straightforward.

Sit-Ups

It strengthens your core muscles, improves back pain problems, and balance. Performing simple sit-ups should do the job. You should feel the sensation in your core muscles.

Chapter 3

WHAT FOODS CAN BE EATEN IN THE KETO DIET AND WHY

Now that we have gotten to the exciting part, it is time to learn what you can and cannot eat while following your new diet. Up until this point, you have most likely followed the food pyramid stating the importance of fruits and vegetables. While they are still going to be important for vitamins and nutrients, you are going to have to be selective. Below, you will find a complete list of foods you get to enjoy on the ketogenic diet!

Keto-Friendly Vegetables

Vegetables can be tricky when you are first starting the ketogenic diet. Some vegetables hold more carbohydrates than others. The simple rule that you need to remember is above the ground is good; below the ground is bad — got that?

Some popular above-ground vegetables you should consider for your diet (starting from the least carbs to the most carbs) include:

- Spinach
- Lettuce
- Avocado
- Asparagus
- Olives
- Cucumber
- Tomato
- Eggplant
- Cabbage
- Zucchini
- Cauliflower
- Kale
- Green Beans
- Broccoli
- Peppers
- Brussel Sprouts

And the below-ground vegetables you should avoid include:

- Carrots
- Onion
- Parsnip
- Beetroot
- Rutabaga
- Potato

- Sweet Potato

Every food that you put on your plate is comprised of three macronutrients: fat, protein, and carbohydrates. This will be an important lesson to learn before you begin your new diet, so be sure to take your time learning how to calculate them.

The golden rule is that meat and dairy are mostly made from protein and fat. Vegetables are mostly carbohydrates. Remember that while following the ketogenic diet, less than 5% of your calories need to come from carbohydrates. This is probably one of the trickiest tasks to get down when you are first getting started; there are hidden carbs everywhere! You will be amazed at how fast 20 g of carbs will go in a single day, much less a single meal!

When you are first getting started, you may want to dip your toes into the carb-cutting. As a rule, vegetables that have less than 5 net carbs can be eaten fairly freely. To make them a bit more ketogenic, I suggest putting butter on your vegetables to get a source of fat into your meal.

If you still struggle at the store, figuring out which vegetables are ketogenic, look for vegetables with leaves. Vegetables that have left are typically spinach and lettuce, both that are keto-friendly. Another rule to follow is to look for green vegetables. Generally, green vegetables like green bell peppers and green cabbage are going to be lower in carbs!

Keto-Friendly Fruits

Much like with the vegetables, some berries and fruits contain hidden carbs. As a general rule, the larger the amount of fruit, the more sugar it contains; this is why fruit is seen as nature's candy! On the ketogenic diet, that is a no go. While berries are going to be okay in moderation, the best is you leave the other fruits out for best results.

You may be thinking to yourself; I need to eat fruits for nutrients! The truth is, you can get the same nutrients from vegetables, costing you fewer carbohydrates on the ketogenic diet. While eating some berries every once in a while won't knock you out of ketosis, it is good to see how they affect you. But, if you feel like indulging in fruit as a treat, you can try some of the following:

- Raspberries
- Blackberries
- Strawberries
- Plum
- Kiwi
- Cherries
- Blueberries

- Clementine
- Cantaloupe
- Peach

Keto-Friendly Meat

On the ketogenic diet, meat is going to become a staple for you! When you are selecting your meats, try to stick with organic, grass-fed, and unprocessed. What I do want you to keep in mind is that the ketogenic diet is not meant to be high in protein, it is meant to be high in fat. People often link the ketogenic diet to a high meat diet, and that simply is not true. As you begin your diet, there is no need to have excess amounts of meat or protein. If you do have excess protein, it is going to be converted to glucose, knocking you right out of ketosis.

There are several different proteins that you will be able to enjoy while following the ketogenic diet. When it comes to beef, you will want to try your best to stick with the fattier cuts. Some of the better cuts would include ground beef, roast, veal, and steak. If poultry is more your style, look for the darker, fattier meats. Some good options for poultry selection would be wild game, turkey, duck, quail, and good old-fashioned chicken. Other options include:

- Pork Loin

- Tenderloin
- Pork Chops
- Ham
- Bacon

On your new diet, you will also be able to enjoy several different seafood dishes! At the store, you will want to look for wild-caught sources. Some of the better options include mahi-mahi, catfish, cod, halibut, trout, sardines, salmon, tuna, and mackerel. If shellfish is more your style, you get to enjoy lobster, muscles, crab, clams, and even oysters!

Keep in mind that when selecting your meats, try to avoid the cured and processed meats. These items, such as jerky, hot dogs, salami, and pepperoni, have many artificial ingredients, additives, and unnecessary sugars that will keep you from reaching ketosis. You know the better options now, stick with them!

Keto-Friendly Nuts

As you begin the ketogenic diet, there is a common misconception that you will now be able to eat as many nuts as you would like because they are high in fat. While you can enjoy a healthy serving of nuts, it is possible to go too nuts on nuts.

Much like with the fruits and the vegetables, you would be surprised to learn that there are hidden carbohydrates here, too!

The lowest carb nuts you are going to find include macadamia nuts, brazil nuts, and pecans. These are fairly low in carbohydrates and can be enjoyed freely while following the ketogenic diet. These are all great options if you are looking for a healthy, ketogenic snack or something to toss in your salad.

When you are at the shop, you will want to avoid the nuts that have been treated with glazes and sugars. All of these extra add sugar and carbohydrates, which you are going to want to avoid. The higher carb nuts include cashews, pistachios, almonds, pine, and peanuts. These nuts can be enjoyed in moderation, but it would be better to avoid.

The issue with eating nuts is that it is easy to overindulge in them. While they are technically keto-friendly, they still contain a high number of calories. With that in mind, you should only be eating when you are hungry and need energy. On the ketogenic diet, you will want to avoid snacking between meals. You don't need the nuts, but they taste good! If you want to lose weight, put the nuts down, and stick to a healthier snack instead.

Keto-Friendly Snacks

On the topic of snacks, let's take a look at keto-friendly ones to have instead of a handful of nuts! Before we begin, keep in mind that if you are looking to lose weight, you will want to avoid snacking when possible. In the beginning, it may be tougher, but as you adapt to the keto diet, your meals should keep your hunger at bay for much longer.

If you are looking for something small to take the edge off your hunger pangs, look for easy whole foods, some of these basics would include eggs, cheese, cold cuts, avocados, and even olives. As long as you have these basics in your fridge, it should stop you from reaching for the high-carb foods.

If you are looking for a snack with more of a crunch, vegetable sticks are always a great option! There are plenty of dipping sauces to add fat to your meal, as well. On top of that, pork rinds are a delicious, zero-carb treat. Beef jerky is also a good option, as long as you are aware of how many carbohydrates are in a commercial package.

With the good options in mind, it's always good to take a look at the bad. When you are snacking, avoid the high-carb fruits, the coffee with creamer, and the sugar-juices. Before you started the ketogenic diet, these were probably the easy option. You'll also want to avoid the obvious candy, chips, and donuts. Just remember when you are selecting your foods, ask if it is fueling you or not.

Keto-Friendly Oils, Sauces, and Fats

On the ketogenic diet, the key to getting enough fat into your diet is going to depend on the sauces and oils you use with your cooking. When you put enough fat into your meals, this is what is going to keep you satisfied after every meal. The secret here is to be careful with the labels. You may be surprised to learn that some of your favorite condiments may have hidden sugars (looking at you, ketchup).

While you are going to have to be a bit more careful about your condiments, you can never go wrong with butter! Up until this point, you have probably been encouraged to consume a low-fat diet. Now, I want you to embrace the fat! You can put butter in absolutely anything! Put butter on your vegetables, stick it in your coffee and get creative!

Oils, on the other hand, can be a bit more complicated. You see, natural oils such as fish oil, sesame oil, almond oil, ghee, pure olive oil, and even peanut oil can be used on absolutely anything. What you want to avoid are the oils that have been created in the past sixty years or so. The oils you'll want to avoid include soy oil, corn oil, sunflower oil, and any vegetable oil. Unfortunately, these oils have been highly processed and may hinder your process.

Stick with these for your diet instead:

- Butter
- Vinaigrette
- Coconut Oil
- Mayo
- Mustard
- Guacamole
- Heavy Cream
- Thousand Island Dressing
- Salsa
- Blue Cheese Dressing
- Ranch Dip
- Pesto

When it comes to dairy, high fat is going to be your best option. Cheese and butter are great options but keep the yogurts in moderation. When it comes to milk, you will want to avoid that as there is extra sugar in milk. If you enjoy heavy cream, this can be excellent for your cooking but should be used sparingly in your coffee.

Keto-Friendly Beverage

Remember that staying hydrated, especially when you are first starting your new diet, is going to be vital! Your safest bet is to always stick with water. Whether you like your water sparkling or flat, this is always going to be a zero-carb option. If you are struggling with a headache or the keto fly, remember that you can always throw a dash of salt in there.

Chapter 4

WHAT FOODS TO AVOID IN THE KETO DIET AND WHY?

Because the diet is a keto, that means you need to avoid high-carbs food. Some of the food you avoid is even healthy, but it just contains too many carbs. Here is a list of typical food you should limit or avoid altogether.

Bread and Grains

No matter what form bread takes, they still pack a lot of carbs. The same applies to wholegrain as well because they are made from refined flour. So, if you want to eat bread, it is best to make keto variants at home instead.

Grains such as rice, wheat, and oats pack a lot of carbs as well. So, limit or avoid that as well.

Fruits

Fruits are healthy for you. The problem is that some of those foods pack quite a lot of carbs such as banana, raisins, dates, mango, and pear. As a general rule, avoid sweet and dried fruits.

Vegetables

Vegetables are just as healthy for your body. For one, they make you feel full for longer, so they help suppress your appetite. But that also means you need to avoid or limit vegetables that are high in starch because they have more carbs than fiber. That includes corn, potato, sweet potato, and beets.

Pasta

As with any other convenient food, pasta is rich in carbs. So, spaghetti or any different types of pasta are not recommended when you are on your keto diet.

Cereal

Cereal is also a considerable offender because sugary breakfast cereals pack a lot of carbs. That also applies to "healthy cereals." Just because they use other words to describe their product does not mean that you should believe them. That also applies to oatmeal, whole-grain cereals, etc.

Beer

In reality, you can drink most alcoholic beverages in moderation without fear. Beer is an exception to this rule because it packs a lot of carbs. Carbs in beers or other liquid are considered liquid carbs, and they are even more dangerous than substantial carbs.

Sweetened Yogurt

Yogurt is very healthy because it is tasty and does not have that many carbs. The problem comes when you consume yogurt variants rich in carbs such as fruit-flavored, low-fat, sweetened, or nonfat yogurt. A single serving of sweetened yogurt contains as many carbs as a single serving of dessert.

Juice

Fruit juices are perhaps the worst beverage you can put into your system when you are on a keto diet. Another problem is that the brain does not process liquid carbs the same way as stable carbs. Substantial carbs can help suppress appetite, but liquid carbs will only put your need into overdrive.

Low-fat and fat-free salad dressings

If you have to buy salads, keep in mind that commercial sauces pack more carbs than you think, especially the fat-free and low-fat variants.

Beans and Legumes

These are also very nutritious as they are rich in fiber. However, they are also rich in carbs. You may enjoy a small amount of them when you are on your keto diet, but don't exceed your carb limit.

Sugar

We mean sugar in any form, including honey. Foods that contain lots of sugar, such as cookies, candies, and cake, are forbidden on a keto diet or any other form of diet that is designed to lose weight. When you are on a keto diet, you need to keep in mind that your diet consists of food that is rich in fiber and nutritious. So, sugar is out of the question.

Chips and Crackers

These two are some of the most popular snacks. Some people did not realize that one packet of chips contains several servings and should not be all eaten in one go. The carbs can add up very quickly if you do not watch what you eat.

Milk

Milk also contains a lot of carbs on its own. Therefore, avoid it if you can even though milk is a good source of many nutrients such as calcium, potassium, and other B vitamins.

Gluten-Free Baked Goods

Gluten-free diets are trendy nowadays, but what many people don't seem to realize is that they pack quite a lot of carbs. That includes gluten-free bread, muffins, and other baked products. In reality, they contain even more carbs than their glutinous variant.

Chapter 5

DOES KETO DIET HAVE SIDE EFFECTS?

It would be very irresponsible of me if I only tell you all the good things about the Ketogenic Diet and ignore the side effects. The truth is that there are negative effects that could happen once you start the Ketogenic Diet – but that's actually true for all of them! All types of diet have negative effects to start with because your body has gotten used to bad habits. Once you make the shift to a more positive way of eating, the body sort of goes on a rebellious phase so it feels like everything is going wrong. For example, a person who used to eat lots of sugar in a day can have severe headaches once they start to avoid sugar. This is a withdrawal symptom and tells you that your diet is actually making positive changes to the body – albeit it takes a little bit of pain on your part.

So, what can one expect when they make that change towards a healthy Ketogenic Diet? Here are some of the things to expect and of course – how to troubleshoot these problems.

Keto Breath

One of the most common side effects of a keto diet is bad breath. Not everyone who adopts the keto diet experiences this problem, but it is common. Bad breath comes as a result of internal metabolism processes. Your liver metabolizes the massive amounts of fat you are consuming and then converts them to ketone bodies such as acetone. These ketone bodies are broken down into smaller organizations and are then circulated inside your body. As the ketone bodies circulate, it gets into your lungs through the diffusion process, and eventually, it is exerted out through your breath.

How to Overcome Keto Breath?

You can control bad keto breath by increasing water intake. You can also get rid of this problem by practicing good oral hygiene like regularly brushing your teeth. Alternatively, you can mask ketosis odor using mints and gums. It is also advisable to eat slightly more carbs and less protein if you have this problem.

Keto Flu

You may experience symptoms resembling those of flu, especially during your first days on a keto diet. Such symptoms include aches, fatigue, cramping, skin rash, and diarrhea. The side effects are caused by dehydration as a result of your body losing a lot of water and electrolytes.

When your body uses fat to fuel its functions instead of using protein, you tend to lose more water and electrolytes through urination. The loss of water and electrolytes is accelerated further by the low insulin levels and muscle glycogen that accompanies the keto diet.

Besides, most keto diets consist of food with little water and potassium levels, further accelerating the loss of body water and electrolytes.

How to Overcome Keto Flu?

You can handle keto flu by drinking much water. You can also eat lots of soup. If you get enough rest, you will give your body enough energy to fight the flu on its own.

You need to lower the effects of keto flu by getting enough sleep. You can also drink much water to minimize the impact of keto flu. There are also some supplements found in natural sources like organic coffee or matcha tea that could help you overcome the flu. Make a point to get enough salts and electrolytes, too.

Fatigue

You may experience extreme feelings of tiredness once you adopt a keto diet. Fatigue is caused by a lack of glucose reaching your brain. Although this side effect will last for a few days, it could still cause much discomfort and worry on your part.

How to Overcome Keto Fatigue?

Drink much water and get enough rest. You can also avoid engaging in strenuous exercises. You can also eat healthy carbs to give you the extra energy your body needs.

GI Side Effects

Keto diet can also harm your digestive system over the long term. Keto diet has been thought to cause some stomach problems such as constipation high cholesterol levels, diarrhea, kidneys stones, and vomiting.

You may also experience abnormal stomach gas due to the sugar alcohols found in some keto diets, for example, the sugars found in some processed foods. The higher the amount of food you eat, the higher the impact of the side effects on you.

How to Control GI Problems When You Are on a Keto Diet?

Drink lots of water and eat high fiber foods such as fruits and vegetables to encourage the growth of beneficial bacteria in your GI system. Make it a habit of exercising regularly.

Weakened Immune System

Keto diets can also weaken the immune systems of some people. Studies suggest that keto foods could cause a condition called dysbiosis. Dysbiosis occurs when the balance of helpful and harmful bacteria is altered in your GI tract. The disruption is caused by the consumption of highly saturated fats and low fiber levels in your digestive system.

When you ingest diets with little prebiotic fiber, the number of beneficial bacteria decreases substantially in your digestive system. Your GI tract is the backbone of your immune system, and any compromise to it could have a negative impact on the immune functions leading to exposure to chronic diseases.

How to Avoid Weakened Immune System When on a Keto Diet?

Incorporate workouts to your keto diet. You can also eat high fiber food, such as fruits and vegetables. Also, ensure you drink lots of water.

Vitamin and Other Mineral Deficiencies

If you are on the keto diet, you may not receive enough vitamins and minerals needed for your body to function normally. Plant-based minerals such as calcium and vitamin D may not be present in your keto diet in the quantities required by your body. If these minerals decrease in your body for long periods, you may stand a high risk of getting lifestyle diseases such as heart failure.

Heart failure comes as a result of the hardening of your heart muscles because of the lack of enough selenium. Selenium is an essential immune-boosting antioxidant usually occurring in plant-based food. Lack of this critical antioxidant causes the hardening of your heart muscles leading to heart failure.

How to Treat the Deficiencies When You Are on a Keto Diet?

Eat lots of fruits and vegetables to get vitamins. You can also use beneficial supplements to treat any deficiencies, which comes with the keto diet.

Increased Risk of Chronic Disease

The Keto diet requires you to put a limit on the number of carbohydrates and protein you consume. When you eat much fat to get enough calories needed by your body, you will be limiting fiber-rich foods such as vegetables, fruits, or legumes. These foods are some of the best sources of immune-boosting nutrients needs by your body to stay healthy. Therefore, when you limit these nutrients in your body, you increase your risk of getting chronic diseases such as diabetes, cancer, high blood pressure.

Studies show that diets that are high in fruits and vegetables can significantly reduce chronic diseases. The more you consume them, the better you are health-wise. When you restrict their consumption, you tend to decrease their beneficial impacts.

How to Reduce the Risk of Chronic Diseases When on Keto Diets?

We'll say it again: drink lots of water. Eat lots of fruits and vegetables. You can also incorporate exercise into your keto diet to get the best results.

Chronic Inflammation

Studies show that when you consume high fats needed for Ketosis, your cholesterol and lipoprotein structure could be significantly altered and will result in inflammation over a while. Inflammation occurs when the cells of your body use much energy to accomplish their normal functioning. Chronic inflammation is also one of the causes of heart diseases.

How to Minimize Chronic Inflammation When on Keto Diets?

You can control the problem of inflammation by eating solid fats and oils. Ensure you also include high fiber foods in your daily intake, like fruits and vegetables.

The Challenge of Weight Cycling

When you restrict your eating diets for an extended period, you may end up gaining too much weight when not dieting, which you then go ahead and lose when on a diet. This process of alternating between weight gain and weight loss is what is referred to as weight cycling. Weight cycling can increase the risk of getting chronic diseases.

How to Control Weight Cycling?

You can control weight cycling by shortening the intervals between dieting and the days you are on free diets. You should gradually increase the amount of food you consume during your free diet days so that your body can have enough time to adjust to the changes in your program.

Chapter 6

BREAKFAST RECIPES

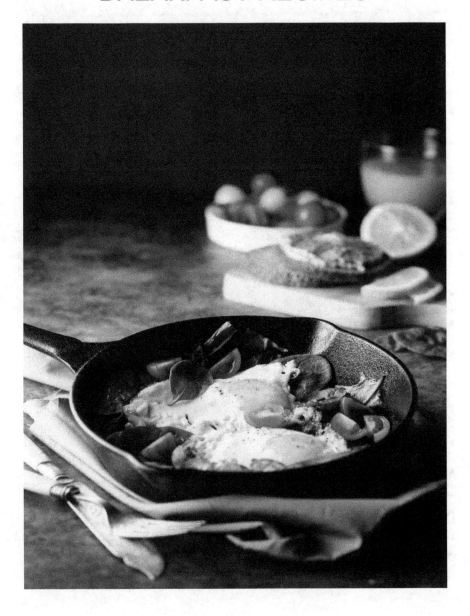

Yogurt Waffles

Prep Time:	Cooking Time:	Servings:
15 min	25 min	4

Ingredients:

- ½ cup golden flax seeds meal
- ½ cup plus 3 tablespoons almond flour
- 1½ tbsp. granulated erythritol
- 1 tbsp. unsweetened vanilla whey protein powder
- ½ tsp. organic powder
- ¼ tsp. xanthan gum
- Salt, to taste
- 1 large organic egg, white and yolk separated
- 1 organic whole egg
- 2 tbsp. unsweetened almond milk
- 1½ tbsp. unsalted butter
- 3 oz. plain Greek yogurt
- ¼ tsp. baking soda.

Directions:

Preheat the waffle iron and then grease it.

In a large bowl, add the flour, erythritol, protein powder, baking soda, baking powder, xanthan gum, salt, and mix until well combined.

In a second small bowl, add the egg white and beat until stiff peaks form.

In a third bowl, add 2 egg yolks, whole egg, almond milk, butter, yogurt and beat until well combined.

Place egg mixture into the bowl of flour mixture and mix until well combined.

Gently, fold in the beaten egg whites.

Place ¼ cup of the mixture into preheated waffle iron and cook for about 4–5 minutes or until golden-brown.

Repeat with the remaining mixture.

Serve warm.

Nutrition:

Calories: 250 kcal | Carbs: 3.2 g | Total Carbs: 8.8 g | Fiber: 5.6 g | Sugar: 1.3 g | Protein 8.4 g.

Broccoli Muffins

Prep Time:	Cooking Time:	Servings:
15 min	20 min	5

Ingredients:

- 2 tbsp. unsalted butter
- 6 large organic eggs
- ½ cup heavy whipping cream
- ½ cup Parmesan cheese, grated
- Salt and ground black pepper, to taste
- 1¼ cup broccoli, chopped
- 2 tbsp. fresh parsley, chopped
- ½ cup Swiss cheese, grated.

Directions:

Preheat your oven to 350°F.

Grease a 12-cup muffin tin.

In a bowl, add the eggs, cream, Parmesan cheese, salt, black pepper and beat until well combined.

Divide the broccoli and parsley in the bottom of each prepared muffin cup evenly.

Top with the egg mixture, followed by the Swiss cheese.

Bake for about 20 minutes, rotating the pan once halfway through.

Remove from the oven and place onto a wire rack for about 5 minutes before serving.

Carefully, invert the muffins onto a serving platter and serve warm.

Nutrition:

Calories: 231 kcal | Total Carbs: 2.5 g | Fiber: 0.5 g | Sugar: 0.9 g | Protein: 13.5 g.

Pumpkin Bread

Prep Time:	Cooking Time:	Servings:
15 min	1 h	5

Ingredients:

- 1⅔ cup almond flour
- 1½ tsp. organic baking powder
- ½ tsp. pumpkin pie spice
- ½ tsp. ground cinnamon
- ½ tsp. ground cloves
- ½ tsp. salt
- 8 oz. cream cheese, softened
- 6 organic eggs, divided
- 1 tbsp. coconut flour
- 1 cup powdered erythritol, divided
- 1 tsp. stevia powder, divided
- 1 tsp. organic lemon extract
- 1 cup homemade pumpkin puree
- ½ cup coconut oil, melted

Directions:

Preheat your oven to 325°F.

Lightly, grease 2 bread loaf pans.

In a bowl, place almond flour, baking powder, spices, salt and mix until well combined.

In a second bowl, add the cream cheese, 1 egg, coconut flour, ¼ cup of erythritol, ¼ teaspoon of the stevia and with a wire whisk, beat until smooth.

In a third bowl, add the pumpkin puree, oil, 5 eggs, ¾ cup of the erythritol, ¾ teaspoon of the stevia, and with a wire whisk, beat until well combined.

Add the pumpkin mixture into the bowl of the flour mixture and mix until just combined.

Place about ¼ of the pumpkin mixture into each loaf pan evenly.

Top each pan with the cream cheese mixture evenly, followed by the remaining pumpkin mixture.

Bake for about 50–60 minutes or until a toothpick inserted in the center comes out clean.

Remove the bread pans from oven and place onto a wire rack and let it be for 10 minutes.

With a sharp knife, cut each bread loaf in the desired-sized slices and serve.

Nutrition:

Calories: 216 kcal | Total Carbs: 4.5 g | Fiber: 2 g | Sugar: 1.1 g |
Protein: 3.4 g.

Spinach Artichoke Breakfast Bake

Prep Time:	Cooking Time:	Servings:
15 min	20 min	7

Ingredients:

- ¼ cup milk, fat-free
- ¼ tsp. ground pepper
- ⅓ cup red pepper, diced
- ½ cup feta cheese crumbles
- ½ cup scallions, finely sliced
- ¾ cup canned artichokes, chopped, drained, & patted dry
- 1¼ tsp. kosher salt
- 1 clove garlic, minced
- 1 tbsp. dill, chopped
- 10 oz. spinach, frozen, chopped & drained
- 2 tbsp. parmesan cheese, grated
- 4 large egg whites
- 8 large eggs.

Directions:

Preheat the oven to 375°F and grease a large baking dish with nonstick spray or preferred fat source.

In a small bowl, combine the spinach, artichoke, scallions, garlic, red pepper, and fill.

Combine completely and then pour into the baking dish, spreading into an even layer.

In a mixing bowl, combine eggs, egg whites, salt, pepper, parmesan, and milk.

Whisk until completely combined, then add feta and mix once more.

Pour the egg mixture evenly over the vegetables in the baking dish.

Bake for about 35 minutes, until a butter knife inserted in the center comes out clean.

Allow to cool for about 10 minutes before cutting into eight equal pieces.

Serve warm!

Nutrition:

Calories: 574 kcal | Carbs: 2 g | Fiber: 0.7 g | Sugar: 0.1 g | Protein: 47 g | Fat: 54 g | Sodium: 254 mg.

Granola Bars

Prep Time:	Cooking Time:	Servings:
15 min	20 min	6

Ingredients:

- 2 cups almonds, chopped
- ½ cup pumpkin seeds, raw
- ⅓ cup coconut flakes, unsweetened
- 2 tbsp. hemp seeds
- ¼ cup clear Sukrin Fiber Syrup
- ¼ cup almond butter
- ¼ cup erythritol, powdered, or equal measure of preferred sweetener
- 2 tsp. vanilla extract
- ½ tsp. sea salt.

Directions:

Line a small, square baking dish with parchment paper.

In a mixing bowl, combine almonds, pumpkin seeds, coconut flakes, and hemp seeds. Stir until evenly mixed.

Over medium heat combine the syrup, almond butter, sweetener, salt, and stir until it's smooth and easy to pull the spoon through.

Remove the pan from the heat and stir the vanilla extract into the mixture.

Pour the syrup over the seeds and stir completely.

Pour the mixture into the baking dish and press evenly into one layer and press until the top is even.

Let cool completely and slice into 12 bars.

Nutrition:

Calories: 254 kcal | Carbs: 2 g | Sugar: 0.1 g | Fiber: 0.7 g | Protein: 42.5 g | Fat: 47 g | Sodium: 145 mg

Chapter 7

LUNCH RECIPES

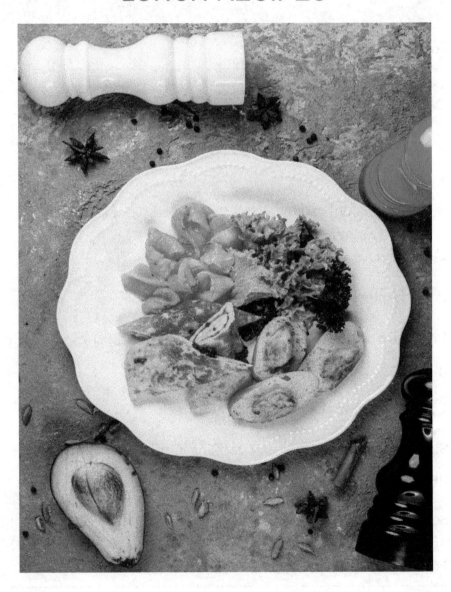

Mushroom & Cauliflower Risotto

Prep Time:	Cooking Time:	Servings:
5 min	10 min	4

Ingredients:

- 1 grated head of cauliflower
- 1 cup vegetable stock
- 9 oz. chopped mushrooms
- 2 tbsp. butter
- 1 cup coconut cream.

Directions:

Pour the stock in a saucepan. Boil and set aside.

Prepare a skillet with butter and sauté the mushrooms until golden.

Grate and stir in the cauliflower and stock.

Simmer and add the cream, cooking until the cauliflower is al dente.

Serve.

Nutrition:

Calories: 186 kcal | Carbs: 4 g | Protein: 1 g | Fats: 17 g.

Pita Pizza

Prep Time:	Cooking Time:	Servings:
15 min	10 min	2

Ingredients:

- ½ cup marinara sauce
- 1 low-carb pita
- 2 oz. cheddar cheese
- 14 slices pepperoni
- 1 oz. roasted red peppers.

Directions:

Program the oven temperature setting to 450°F.

Slice the pita in half and place onto a foil-lined baking tray.

Rub with a bit of oil and toast for one to two minutes.

Pour the sauce over the bread.

Sprinkle using the cheese and other toppings.

Bake until the cheese melts (5 minutes).Cool thoroughly.

Nutrition:

Calories: 250 kcal | Carbs: 4 g | Protein: 13 g | Fats: 19 g.

Italian Style Halibut Packets

Ingredients:

- 2 cups cauliflower florets
- 1 cup roasted red pepper strips
- ½ cup sliced sun-dried tomatoes
- 4 (4-ounce) halibut fillets
- ¼ cup chopped fresh basil
- 1 lemon juice
- ¼ cup good-quality olive oil
- Sea salt, for seasoning
- Freshly ground black pepper, for seasoning.

Directions:

Preheat the oven. Set the oven temperature to 400°F.

Make the packets.

Divide the cauliflower, red pepper strips, and sun-dried tomato between the four pieces of foil, placing the vegetables in the middle of each piece.

Top each pile with one halibut fillet and top each fillet with equal amounts of the basil, lemon juice, and olive oil.

Fold and crimp the foil to form sealed packets of fish and vegetables and place them on the baking sheet.

Bake. Bake the packets for about 20 minutes, until the fish flakes with a fork.

Be careful of the steam when you open the packet!

Serve. Transfer the vegetables and halibut to four plates, season with salt and pepper, and serve immediately.

Nutrition:

Calories: 313 kcal | Fat: 14.1 g | Carbs: 3.2 g | Fiber: 10.4 g | Protein: 15.4 g.

Taco Casserole

Prep Time:	Cooking Time:	Servings:
10 min	20 min	8

Ingredients:

- 1½ to 2 lb. ground turkey or beef
- 2 tbsp. taco seasoning
- 8 oz. shredded cheddar cheese
- 1 cup salsa
- 16 oz. cottage cheese.

Directions:

Heat the oven to reach 400 °F.

Combine the taco seasoning and ground meat in a casserole dish.

Bake it for 20 minutes.

Combine the salsa and both kinds of cheese. Set aside for now.

Carefully transfer the casserole dish from the oven.

Drain away the cooking juices from the meat.

Break the meat into small pieces and mash with a masher or fork.

Sprinkle with cheese.

Bake in the oven for 15 to 20 more minutes until the top is browned.

Nutrition:

Calories: 367 kcal | Carbs: 6 g | Protein: 45 g | Fats: 18 g.

Beef Wellington

Prep Time:	Cooking Time:	Servings:
20 min	40 min	4

Ingredients:

- 2 (4-ounce) grass-fed beef tenderloin steaks, halved
- Salt and ground black pepper, as required
- 1 tbsp. butter
- 1 cup mozzarella cheese, shredded
- ½ cup almond flour
- 4 tbsp. liver pate.

Directions:

Preheat your oven to 400°F.

Grease a baking sheet.

Season the steaks with pepper and salt.

Sear the beef steaks for about 2–3 minutes per side.

In a microwave-safe bowl, add the mozzarella cheese and microwave for about 1 minute.

Remove from the microwave and stir in the almond flour until a dough forms.

Place the dough between 2 parchment paper pieces and, with a rolling pin, roll to flatten it.

Remove the upper parchment paper piece.

Divide the rolled dough into four pieces.

Place one tablespoon of pate onto each dough piece and top with one steak piece.

Cover each steak piece with dough completely.

Arrange the covered steak pieces onto the prepared baking sheet in a single layer.

Baking time: 20-30 minutes.

Serve warm.

Nutrition:

Calories: 412 kcal | Fat: 15.6g | Carbs: 4.9 g | Fiber: 9.1g | Protein: 18.5g.

Keto Croque Monsieur

Prep Time:	Cooking Time:	Servings:
5 min	7 min	2

Ingredients:

- 2 eggs
- ¾ oz. of grated cheese
- ¾ oz. of ham 1 large slice
- 3 tbsp. of cream
- 3 tbsp. of mascarpone
- 1 oz. of butter
- Pepper and salt
- Basil leaves, optional, to garnish.

Directions:

Carefully crack eggs in a neat bowl, add some salt and pepper.

Add the cream, mascarpone, grated cheese, and stir together.

Melt the butter over medium heat. The butter must not turn brown.

Once the butter has melted, set the heat to low.

Add half of the omelette mixture to the frying pan and then immediately place the slice of ham on it.

Now pour the rest of the omelette mixture over the ham and then immediately put a lid on it.

Allow it to fry for 2-3 minutes over low heat until the top is slightly firmer.

Slide the omelette onto the lid to turn the omelette.

Then put the omelette back in the frying pan to fry for another 1-2 minutes on the other side (still on low heat), then put the lid back on the pan.

Don't let the omelette cook for too long!

It does not matter if it is still liquid.

Garnish with a few basil leaves if necessary.

Nutrition:

Calories: 479 kcal | Protein: 16 g | Fats: 45 g | Carbs: 4 g.

Keto Wraps with Cream Cheese and Salmon

Prep Time:	Cooking Time:	Servings:
5 min	10 min	2

Ingredients:

- 3 oz. of cream cheese
- 1 tbsp. of dill or other fresh herbs
- 1 oz. of smoked salmon
- 1 egg
- ½ oz. of butter
- Pinch of cayenne pepper
- Pepper and salt.

Directions:

Beat the egg well in a bowl. With 1 egg, you can make two thin wraps in a small frying pan.

Melt the butter over medium heat in a small frying pan.

Once the butter has melted, add half of the beaten egg to the pan.

Move the pan back and forth so that the entire bottom is covered with a very thin layer of egg. Turn down the heat!

Carefully loosen the egg on the edges with a silicone spatula and turn the wafer-thin omelets as soon as the egg is no longer dripping (about 45 seconds to 1 minute).

You can do this by sliding it onto a lid or plate and then sliding it back into the pan.

Let the other side be cooked for about 30 seconds and then remove from the pan.

The omelets must be nice and light yellow.

Repeat for the rest of the beaten egg.

Once the omelets are ready, let them cool on a cutting board or plate and make the filling.

Cut the dill into small pieces and put in a bowl

Add the cream cheese, the salmon cut into small pieces, and mix together. Add a tiny bit of cayenne pepper and mix well. Taste immediately and then season with salt and pepper.

Spread a layer on the wrap and roll it up. Cut the wrap in half and keep in the fridge until you are ready to eat it.

Nutrition:

Calories: 237 kcal | Carbs: 14.7 g | Protein: 15 g | Fat: 5 g.

Sesame Pork with Green Beans

Prep Time:	Cooking Time:	Servings:
5 min	10 min	2

Ingredients:

- 2 boneless pork chops
- Pink Himalayan salt
- Freshly ground black pepper
- 2 tbsp. toasted sesame oil, divided
- 2 tbsp. soy sauce
- 1 tsp. Sriracha sauce
- 1 cup fresh green beans.

Directions:

On a cutting board, pat the pork chops dry with a paper towel. Slice the chops into strips and season with pink Himalayan salt and pepper.

In a large skillet over medium heat, heat one tablespoon of sesame oil.

Add the pork strips and cook them for 7 minutes, stirring occasionally.

In a small bowl, mix the remaining one tablespoon of sesame oil, the soy sauce, and the Sriracha sauce. Pour into the skillet with the pork.

Add the green beans to the skillet, reduce the heat to medium-low, and simmer for 3 to 5 minutes.

Divide the pork, green beans, and sauce between two wide, shallow bowls and serve.

Nutrition:

Calories: 387 kcal | Fat: 15.1 g | Carbs: 4.1 g | Fiber: 10 g | Protein: 18.1 g

Pan-Seared Cod with Tomato Hollandaise

Prep Time:	Cooking Time:	Servings:
10 min	10 min	4

Ingredients:

- Pan-Seared Cod
- 1 pound (4-fillets) wild Alaskan Cod
- 1 tbsp. salted butter
- 1 tbsp. olive oil
- Tomato Hollandaise
- 3 large egg yolks
- 3 tbsp. warm water
- 8 oz. salted butter, melted
- ¼ tsp. salt
- ¼ tsp. black pepper
- 2 tbsp. tomato paste
- 2 tbsp. fresh lemon juice.

Directions:

Season both sides of the code fillet without salt, the salt will be added in the last.

Heat a skillet over medium heat and coat with olive oil and butter.

When the butter heats up, place the cod fillet in the skillet and sear on both sides for 2-3 minutes. Baste the fish fillet with the oil and butter mixture.

You will know that the cod cooked when it easily flakes when poked with a fork.

Melt the butter in the microwave.

In a double boil, beat egg yolks with warm water until thick and creamy and start forming soft peaks. Remove the double boil from the heat, gradually adding the melted butter and stirring.

Season.

Mix in the tomato paste. Stir to combine. Pour in the water and lemon juice to lighten the sauce texture.

Nutrition:

Calories: 356 | Fat: 16.1 g | Carbs: 3.1 g | Fiber: 12.3 g | Protein: 18.4 g.

Creamy Scallops

Prep Time:	Cooking Time:	Servings:
10 min	10 min	4

Ingredients:

- 1 lb. scallops, rinse and pat dry
- 1 tsp. fresh parsley, chopped
- ⅛ tsp. cayenne pepper
- 2 tbsp. white wine
- ¼ cup water
- 3 tbsp. heavy cream
- 1 tsp. garlic, minced
- 1 tbsp. butter, melted
- 1 tbsp. olive oil
- Pepper
- Salt.

Direction:

Season scallops with pepper and salt.

Heat butter and oil in a pan over medium heat.

Add scallops and sear until browned from both sides. Transfer scallops on a plate.

Add garlic in the same pan and sauté for 30 seconds.

Add water, heavy cream, wine, cayenne pepper, and salt. Stir well and cook until sauce thickens.

Return scallops to pan and stir well.

Garnish with parsley and serve.

Nutrition:

Calories: 202 kcal | Fat: 11.4 g | Cholesterol: 60 mg | Carbs: 3.5 g | Sugar: 0.1 g | Protein: 19.4 g.

Perfect Pan-Seared Scallops

Prep Time:	Cooking Time:	Servings:
10 min	4 min	4

Ingredients:

- 1 lb. scallops, rinse and pat dry
- 1 tbsp. olive oil
- 2 tbsp. butter
- Pepper
- Salt.

Direction:

Season scallops with pepper and salt.

Heat butter and oil in a pan over medium heat.

Add scallops and sear for 2 minutes then turn to the other side and cook for 2 minutes more.

Serve and enjoy.

Nutrition:

Calories: 181 kcal | Fat: 10.1 g | Cholesterol: 53 mg | Carbs: 2.7 g | Sugar: 0 g | Protein: 19.1 g.

Easy Baked Shrimp Scampi

Prep Time:	Cooking Time:	Servings:
10 min	10 min	4

Ingredients:

- 2 lb. shrimp, peeled
- ¾ cup olive oil
- 2 tsp. dried oregano
- 1 tbsp. garlic, minced
- ½ cup fresh lemon juice
- ¼ cup butter, sliced
- Pepper
- Salt.

Directions:

Preheat the oven to 350°F.

Add shrimp in a baking dish.

In a bowl, whisk together lemon juice, oregano, garlic, oil, pepper, salt, and pour over shrimp.

Add butter on top of shrimp.

Bake in preheated oven for 10 minutes or until shrimp is cooked.

Serve and enjoy.

Nutrition:

Calories: 708 kcal | Fat: 53.5 g | Cholesterol: 508 mg | Carbs: 5.3 g | Sugar: 0.7 g | Protein: 52.2 g.

Delicious Blackened Shrimp

Prep Time:	Cooking Time:	Servings:
10 min	5 min	4

Ingredients:

- 1½ lbs. shrimp, peeled
- 1 tbsp. garlic, minced
- 1 tbsp. olive oil
- 1 tsp. garlic powder
- 1 tsp. dried oregano
- 1 tsp. cumin
- 1 tbsp. paprika
- 1 tbsp. chili powder
- Pepper
- Salt.

Direction:

In a mixing bowl, mix together garlic powder, oregano, cumin, paprika, chili powder, pepper, and salt.

Add shrimp and mix until well coated. Set aside for 30 minutes.

Heat oil in a pan over medium-high heat.

Add shrimp and cook for 2 minutes. Turn shrimp and cook for 2 minutes more.

Add garlic and cook for 30 seconds.

Serve and enjoy.

Nutrition:

Calories 252 kcal | Fat: 7.1 g | Cholesterol: 358 mg | Carbs: 6.3 g | Sugar: 0.5 g | Protein: 39.6 g.

Signature Italian Pork Dish

Prep Time:	Cooking Time:	Servings:
15 min	15 min	6

Ingredients:

- 2 lb. pork tenderloins, cut into 1½-inch pieces
- ¼ cup almond flour
- 1 tsp. garlic salt
- Freshly ground black pepper, to taste
- 2 tbsp. butter
- ½ cup homemade chicken broth
- ⅓ cup balsamic vinegar
- 1 tbsp. capers
- 2 tsp. fresh lemon zest, grated finely.

Direction:

In a large bowl, add the pork pieces, flour, garlic salt, black pepper, and toss to coat well.

Remove pork pieces from bowl and shake off excess flour mixture.

In a large skillet, melt the butter over medium-high heat and cook the pork pieces for about 2-3 minutes per side.

Add broth and vinegar and bring to a gentle boil.

Reduce the heat to medium and simmer for about 3-4 minutes.

With a slotted spoon, transfer the pork pieces onto a plate.

In the same skillet, add the capers, lemon zest, and simmer for about 3-5 minutes or until the desired thickness of sauce.

Pour sauce over pork pieces and serve.

Nutrition:

Calories: 373 kcal | Carbs: 1.8 g | Fiber: 0.7 g | Sugar: 0.4 g | Protein: 46.7 g | Fat: 18.6 g | Sodium: 231 mg.

Flavor Packed Pork Loin

Prep Time:	Cooking Time:	Servings:
15 min	1 h	6

Ingredients:

- ⅓ cup low-sodium soy sauce
- ¼ cup fresh lemon juice
- 2 tsp. fresh lemon zest, grated
- 1 tbs. fresh thyme, finely chopped
- 2 tbsp. fresh ginger, grated
- 2 garlic cloves, chopped finely
- 2 tbsp. Erythritol
- Freshly ground black pepper, to taste
- ½ tsp. cayenne pepper
- 2 lb. boneless pork loin.

Direction:

For pork marinade: in a large baking dish, add all the ingredients except pork loin and mix until well combined.

Add the pork loin and coat with the marinade generously.

Refrigerate for about 24 hours.

Preheat the oven to 400°F.

Remove the pork loin from marinade and arrange it into a baking dish.

Cover the baking dish and bake for about 1 hour.

Remove from the oven and place the pork loin onto a cutting board.

With a piece of foil, cover each loin for at least 10 minutes before slicing.

With a sharp knife, cut the pork loin into desired size slices and serve.

Nutrition:

Calories: 230 kcal | Carbs: 3.2 g | Fiber: 0.6 g | Sugar: 1.2 g | Protein: 40.8 g | Fat: 5.6 g | Sodium: 871 mg

Chapter 8

DINNER RECIPES

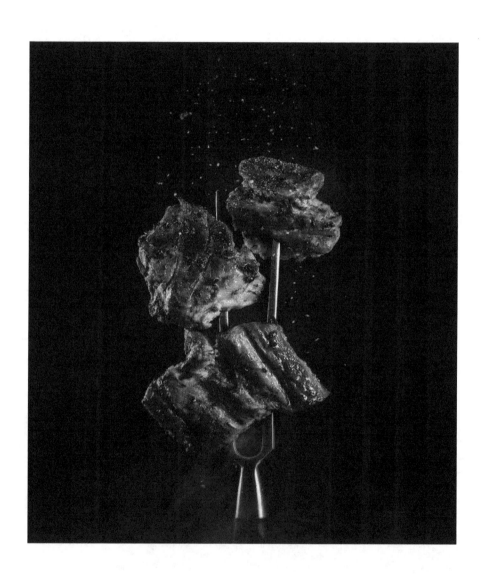

Korma Curry

Prep Time:	Cooking Time:	Servings:
10 min	25 min	6

Ingredients:

- 3-pound chicken breast, skinless, boneless
- 1 tsp. garam masala
- 1 tsp. curry powder
- 1 tbsp. apple cider vinegar
- ½ coconut cream
- 1 cup organic almond milk
- 1 tsp. ground coriander
- ¾ tsp. ground cardamom
- ½ tsp. ginger powder
- ¼ tsp. cayenne pepper
- ¾ tsp. ground cinnamon
- 1 tomato, diced
- 1 tsp. avocado oil
- ½ cup of water.

Directions:

Chop the chicken breast and put it in the saucepan.

Add avocado oil and start to cook it over medium heat.

Sprinkle the chicken with garam masala, curry powder, apple cider vinegar, ground coriander, cardamom, ginger powder, cayenne pepper, ground cinnamon, and diced tomato. Mix up the ingredients carefully.

Cook them for 10 minutes.

Add water, coconut cream, and almond milk. Sauté the meat for 10 minutes more.

Nutrition:

Calories: 440 kcal | Fat: 32 g | Fiber: 4 g | Carbs: 28 g | Protein: 8 g.

Creamy Zoodles

Prep Time:	Cooking Time:	Servings:
15 min	10 min	4

Ingredients:

- 1¼ cups heavy whipping cream
- ¼ cup mayonnaise
- Salt and ground black pepper, as required
- 30 oz. zucchini, spiralized with blade C
- 3 oz. Parmesan cheese, grated
- 2 tbsp. fresh mint leaves
- 2 tbsp. butter, melted.

Directions:

The heavy cream must be added to a pan then bring to a boil.

Lower the heat to low and cook until reduced in half.

Put in the pepper, mayo, and salt; cook until mixture is warm enough.

Add the zucchini noodles and gently stir to combine.

Stir in the Parmesan cheese.

Divide the zucchini noodles onto four serving plates and immediately drizzle with the melted butter.

Serve immediately.

Nutrition:

Calories: 241 kcal| Fat: 11.4 g | Fiber: 7.5 g | Carbs: 3.1 g | Protein: 5.1 g.

Cheesy Bacon Squash Spaghetti

Prep Time:	Cooking Time:	Servings:
30 min	50 min	4

Ingredients:

- 2 pounds spaghetti squash
- 2 pounds bacon
- ½ cup of butter
- 2 cups of shredded parmesan cheese
- Salt
- Black pepper.

Directions:

Let the oven preheat to 375°F.

Trim or remove each stem of spaghetti squash, slice into rings no more than an inch wide, and take out the seeds.

Lay the sliced rings down on the baking sheet, bake for 40-45 minutes.

It is ready when the strands separate easily when a fork is used to scrape it. Let it cool.

Cook sliced up bacon until crispy. Take out and let it cool.

Take off the shell on each ring, separate each strand with a fork, and put them in a bowl.

Heat the strands in a microwave to get them warm, then put in butter and stir around till the butter melts.

Pour in parmesan cheese and bacon crumbles and add salt and pepper to your taste. Enjoy.

Nutrition:

Calories: 398 kcal | Fat: 12.5 g | Fiber: 9.4 g | Carbs: 4.1 g | Protein: 5.1 g.

Stuffed Portobello Mushrooms

Prep Time:	Cooking Time:	Servings:
10 min	10 min	4

Ingredients:

- 2 portobello mushrooms
- 1 cup spinach, chopped, steamed
- 2 oz. artichoke hearts, drained, chopped
- 1 tbsp. coconut cream
- 1 tbsp. cream cheese
- 1 tsp. minced garlic
- 1 tbsp. fresh cilantro, chopped
- 3 oz. Cheddar cheese, grated
- ½ tsp. ground black pepper
- 2 tbsp. olive oil
- ½ tsp. salt.

Directions:

Sprinkle mushrooms with olive oil and place in the tray.

Transfer the tray to the preheated to 360°F oven and broil them for 5 minutes.

Meanwhile, blend artichoke hearts, coconut cream, cream cheese, minced garlic, and chopped cilantro.

Add grated cheese to the mixture and sprinkle with ground black pepper and salt.

Fill the broiled mushrooms with the cheese mixture and cook them for 5 minutes more. Serve the mushrooms only hot.

Nutrition:

Calories: 135.2 kcal | Total Fat: 5.5 g | Cholesterol: 16.4 mg | Sodium: 698.1 mg | Potassium: 275.3 mg | Carbs: 8.4 g | Protein: 14.8 g.

Pesto Flavored Steak

Prep Time:	Cooking Time:	Servings:
15 min	17 min	4

Ingredients:

- ¼ cup fresh oregano, chopped
- 1½ tbsp. garlic, minced
- 1 tbsp. fresh lemon peel, grated
- ½ tsp. red pepper flakes, crushed
- Salt and freshly ground black pepper, to taste
- 1 lb. (1-inch thick) grass-fed boneless beef top sirloin steak
- 1 cup pesto
- ¼ cup feta cheese, crumbled.

Direction:

Preheat the gas grill to medium heat. Lightly, grease the grill grate.

In a bowl, add the oregano, garlic, lemon peel, red pepper flakes, salt, black pepper, and mix well.

Rub the garlic mixture onto the steak evenly.

Place the steak onto the grill and cook, covered for about 12-17 minutes, flipping occasionally.

Remove from the grill and place the steak onto a cutting board for about 5 minutes.

With a sharp knife, cut the steak into desired sized slices.

Divide the steak slices and pesto onto serving plates and serve with the topping of the feta cheese.

Nutrition:

Calories: 226 kcal | Carbs: 6.8 g | Sugar: 0.7 g | Fiber: 2.2 g | Protein: 40.5 g | Fat: 7.6 g | Sodium: 579 mg.

Flawless Grilled Steak

Prep Time:	Cooking Time:	Servings:
21 min	10 min	5

Ingredients:

- ½ tsp. dried thyme, crushed
- ½ tsp. dried oregano, crushed
- 1 tsp. red chili powder
- ½ tsp. ground cumin
- ¼ tsp. garlic powder
- Salt and freshly ground black pepper, to taste
- 1½ lb. grass-fed flank steak, trimmed
- ¼ cup Monterrey Jack cheese, crumbled.

Direction:

In a large bowl, add the dried herbs and spices and mix well.

Add the steaks and rub with mixture generously.

Set aside for about 15-20 minutes.

Preheat the grill to medium heat. Grease the grill grate.

Place the steak onto the grill over medium coals and cook for about 17-21 minutes, flipping once halfway through.

Remove the steak from the grill and place onto a cutting board for about 10 minutes before slicing.

With a sharp knife, cut the steak into desired sized slices.

Top with the cheese and serve.

Nutrition:

Calories: 271 kcal | Carbs: 0.7 g | Sugar: 0.1 g | Fiber: 0.3 g | Protein: 38.3 g | Fat: 11.8 g | Sodium: 119 mg.

Brussels Sprouts with Bacon

Prep Time:	Cooking Time:	Servings:
15 min	40 min	6

Ingredients:

- 16 oz. bacon
- 16 oz. Brussel sprouts
- Black pepper.

Directions:

Warm the oven to reach 400°F.

Slice the bacon into small lengthwise pieces. Put the sprouts and bacon with pepper.

Bake within 35 to 40 minutes. Serve.

Nutrition:

Calories: 113 kcal | Carbs: 3.9 g | Protein: 7.9 g | Total Fats: 6.9 g.

Kalua Pork with Cabbage

Prep Time:	Cooking Time:	Servings:
10 min	8 h	4

Ingredients:

- 1-pound boneless pork butt roast
- Pink Himalayan salt
- Freshly ground black pepper
- 1 tbsp. smoked paprika or Liquid Smoke
- ½ cup of water
- ½ head cabbage, chopped.

Directions:

With the crock insert in place, preheat the slow cooker to low.

Generously season the pork roast with pink Himalayan salt, pepper, and smoked paprika.

Place the pork roast in the slow-cooker insert, and add the water.

Cover and cook on low for 7 hours.

Transfer the cooked pork roast to a plate. Put the chopped cabbage in the bottom of the slow cooker, and put the pork roast back in on the cabbage.

Cover and cook the cabbage and pork roast for 1 hour.

Remove the pork roast from the slow cooker and place it on a baking sheet. Use two forks to shred the pork.

Serve the shredded pork hot with the cooked cabbage.

Reserve the liquid from the slow cooker to remoisten the pork and cabbage when reheating leftovers.

Nutrition:

Calories: 451 kcal | Fat: 19.3 g | Carbs: 2.1 g | Fiber: 11.2 g | Protein: 14.3 g.

Coffee BBQ Pork Belly

Prep Time:	Cooking Time:	Servings:
15 min	60 min	4

Ingredients:

- 1½ cup beef stock
- 2 lb. pork belly
- 4 tbsp. olive oil
- Low-carb barbecue dry rub
- 2 tbsp. instant Espresso Powder.

Directions:

Set the oven at 350°F.

Heat-up the beef stock in a small saucepan.

Mix in the dry barbecue rub and espresso powder.

Put the pork belly, skin side up in a shallow dish and drizzle half of the oil over the top.

Put the hot stock around the pork belly. Bake within 45 minutes.

Sear each slice within three minutes per side. Serve.

Nutrition:

Calories: 644 kcal | Carbs: 2.6 g | Protein: 24 g | Total Fats: 68 g.

Garlic & Thyme Lamb Chops

Prep Time:	Cooking Time:	Servings:
15 min	10 min	6

Ingredients:

- 6 - 4 oz. lamb chops
- 4 whole garlic cloves
- 2 thyme sprigs
- 1 tsp. ground thyme
- 3 tbsp. olive oil.

Directions:

Warm-up a skillet. Put the olive oil. Rub the chops with the spices.

Put the chops in the skillet with the garlic and sprigs of thyme.

Sauté within 3 to 4 minutes and serve.

Nutrition:

Calories: 252 kcal | Carbs: 1 g | Protein: 14 g | Fats: 21 g.

Jamaican Jerk Pork Roast

Ingredients:

- 1 tbsp. olive oil
- 4 lb. pork shoulder
- ½ cup beef Broth
- ¼ cup Jamaican Jerk spice blend.

Directions:

Rub the roast well the oil and the jerk spice blend.

Sear the roast on all sides.

Put the beef broth.

Simmer within 4 hours on low.

Shred and serve.

Nutrition:

Calories: 282 kcal | Carbs: 0 g | Protein: 23 g | Fats: 20 g.

Keto Meatballs

Ingredients:

- 1 egg
- ½ cup grated parmesan
- ½ cup shredded mozzarella
- 1 lb. ground beef
- 1 tbsp. garlic.

Directions:

Warm-up the oven to reach 400°F.

Combine all of the fixings. Shape into meatballs.

Bake within 18-20 minutes.

Cool and serve.

Nutrition:

Calories: 153 kcal | Carbs: 0.7 g | Protein: 12.2 g | Fats: 10.9 g.

Mixed Vegetable Patties

Prep Time:	Cooking Time:	Servings:
15 min	10 min	4

Ingredients:

- 1 cup cauliflower florets
- 1 bag vegetables
- 1½ cup Water
- 1 cup flax meal
- 2 tbsp. olive oil.

Directions:

Steam the veggies to the steamer basket within 4 to 5 minutes.

Mash in the flax meal.

Shape into 4 patties.

Cook the patties within 3 minutes per side. Serve.

Nutrition:

Calories: 220 kcal | Carbs: 3 g | Protein: 4 g | Fats: 10 g.

Roasted Leg of Lamb

Ingredients:

- ½ cup reduced-sodium beef broth
- 2 lb. lamb leg
- 6 garlic cloves
- 1 tbsp. rosemary leaves
- 1 tsp. black pepper.

Directions:

Warm-up oven temperature to 400°F.

Put the lamb in the pan and put the broth and seasonings.

Roast 30 minutes and lower the heat to 350°F. Cook within 1 hour.

Cool and serve.

Nutrition:

Calories: 223 kcal | Carbs: 1 g | Protein: 22 g | Fats: 14 g.

Mongolian Beef

Ingredients:

- 1 lb. grass-fed flank steak, cut into thin slices against the grain
- 2 tsp. arrowroot starch
- Salt, to taste
- ¼ cup avocado oil
- 1 (1-inch) piece fresh ginger, grated
- 4 garlic cloves, minced
- ½ tsp. red pepper flakes, crushed
- ¼ cup water
- ⅓ cup low-sodium soy sauce
- 1 tsp. red boat fish sauce
- 3 scallions, sliced
- 1 tsp. sesame seeds.

Direction:

In a bowl, add the steak slices, arrowroot starch, salt, and toss to coat well.

In a larger skillet, heat oil over medium-high heat and cook the steak slices for about 1½ minutes per side.

With a slotted spoon, transfer the steak slices onto a plate.

Drain the oil from the skillet but leaving about 1 tbsp. inside.

In the same skillet, add the ginger, garlic, red pepper flakes, and sauté for about 1 minute.

Add the water, soy sauce, fish sauce, and stir to combine well.

Stir in the cooked steak slices and simmer for about 3 minutes.

Stir in the scallions and simmer for about 2 minutes.

Remove from the heat and serve hot with the garnishing of sesame seeds.

Nutrition:

Calories: 266 kcal | Carbs: 5.7 g | Sugar: 1.7 g | Fiber: 1.2 g | Protein: 34 g | Fat: 11.7 g | Sodium: 1350 mg.

Lettuce Salad

Prep Time:	Cooking Time:	Servings:
10 min	0 min	1

Ingredients:

- 1 cup Romaine lettuce, roughly chopped
- 3 oz. seitan, chopped
- 1 tbsp. avocado oil
- 1 tsp. sunflower seeds
- 1 tsp. lemon juice
- 1 egg, boiled, peeled
- 2 oz. Cheddar cheese, shredded.

Directions:

Place lettuce in the salad bowl. Add chopped seitan and shredded cheese.

Then chop the egg roughly and add in the salad bowl too.

Mix up together lemon juice with the avocado oil.

Sprinkle the salad with the oil mixture and sunflower seeds. Don't stir the salad before serving.

Nutrition:

Calories: 20 kcal | Fat: 0.2 g | Cholesterol: 0 mg | Sodium: 31 mg | Potassium: 241 mg | Carbs: 4.2 g | Protein: 1.2 g.

Grain-Free Creamy Noodles

Prep Time:	Cooking Time:	Servings:
15 min	10 min	4

Ingredients:

- 1¼ cup heavy whipping cream
- ¼ cup mayonnaise
- Salt and freshly ground black pepper, to taste
- 30 oz. zucchini, spiralized with blade
- 4 organic egg yolks
- 3 oz. Parmesan cheese, grated
- 2 tbsp. fresh parsley, chopped
- 2 tbsp. butter, melted.

Direction:

In a pan, add the heavy cream and bring to a boil.

Reduce the heat to low and cook until reduced.

Add the mayonnaise, salt, black pepper, and cook until the mixture is warm enough.

Add the zucchini noodles and gently, stir to combine.

Immediately, remove from the heat.

Place the zucchini noodles mixture onto 4 serving plates evenly and immediately, top with the egg yolks, followed by the parmesan and parsley.

Drizzle with hot melted butter and serve.

Nutrition:

Calories: 427 kcal | Carbs: 9 g | Sugar: 3.8 g | Fiber: 2.4 g | Protein: 13 g | Fat: 39.1 g | Sodium: 412 mg.

Meat-Free Zoodles Stroganoff

Prep Time:	Cooking Time:	Servings:
20 min	12 min	5

Ingredients:

For Mushroom Sauce:

- 1½ tbsp. butter
- 1 large garlic clove, minced
- 1¼ cup fresh button mushrooms, sliced
- ¼ cup homemade vegetable broth
- ¼ cup cream
- Salt and freshly ground black pepper, to taste.

For Zucchini Noodles:

- 3 large zucchinis, spiralized with blade
- ¼ cup fresh parsley leaves, chopped.

Direction:

For mushroom sauce: in a large skillet, melt the butter over medium heat and sauté the garlic for about 1 minute.

Stir in the mushrooms and cook for about 6-8 minutes.

Stir in the broth and cook for about 2 minutes, stirring continuously.

Stir in the cream, salt, and black pepper and cook for about 1 minute.

<u>Meanwhile, for the zucchini noodles:</u> in a large pan of boiling water, add the zucchini noodles and cook for about 2-3 minutes.

With a slotted spoon, transfer the zucchini noodles into a colander and immediately rinse under cold running water.

Drain the zucchini noodles well and transfer onto a large paper towel-lined plate to drain.

Divide the zucchini noodles onto serving plates evenly.

Remove the mushroom sauce from the heat and place over zucchini noodles evenly.

Serve immediately with the garnishing of parsley.

Nutrition:

Calories: 77 kcal | Carbs: 7.9 g | Sugar: 4 g | Fiber: 2.4 g | Protein: 3.4 g | Fat: 4.6 g | Sodium: 120 mg.

Eye-Catching Veggies

Prep Time:	Cooking Time:	Servings:
51 min	20 min	4

Ingredients:

- ¼ cup butter
- 6 scallions, sliced
- 1 lb. fresh white mushrooms, sliced
- 1 cup tomatoes, crushed
- Salt and freshly ground black pepper, to taste
- 2 tbsp. feta cheese, crumbled

Direction:

In a large pan, melt the butter over medium-low heat and sauté the scallion for about 2 minutes.

Add the mushrooms and sauté for about 5-7 minutes.

Stir in the tomatoes and cook for about 8-10 minutes, stirring occasionally.

Stir in the salt and black pepper and remove from the heat.

Serve with the topping of feta.

Nutrition:

Calories: 160 kcal | Carbs: 7.4 g | Sugar: 3.9 g | Fiber: 2.3 g | Protein: 5.5 g | Fat: 13.5 g | Sodium: 211 mg.

Chicken Schnitzel

Prep Time:	Cooking Time:	Servings:
15 min	15-22 min	4

Ingredients:

- 1 tbsp. chopped fresh parsley
- 4 garlic cloves, minced
- 1 tbsp. plain vinegar
- 1 tbsp. coconut aminos
- 2 tsp. sugar-free maple syrup
- 2 tsp. chili pepper
- Salt and black pepper to taste
- 6 tbsp. coconut oil
- 1 lb. asparagus, hard stems removed
- 4 chicken breasts, skin-on and boneless
- 2 cups grated Mexican cheese blend
- 1 tbsp. mixed sesame seeds
- 1 cup almond flour
- 4 eggs, beaten
- 6 tbsp. avocado oil
- 1 tsp. chili flakes for garnish

Directions:

In a bowl, whisk the parsley, garlic, vinegar, coconut aminos, maple syrup, chili pepper, salt, and black pepper. Set aside.

Heat the coconut oil in a large skillet and stir-fry the asparagus for 8 to 10 minutes or until tender. Remove the asparagus into a large bowl and toss with the vinegar mixture. Set aside for serving.

Cover the chicken breasts in plastic wraps and use a meat tenderizer to pound the chicken until flattened to 2-inch thickness gently.

On a plate, mix the Mexican cheese blend and sesame seeds. Dredge the chicken pieces in the almond flour, dip in the egg on both sides, and generously coat in the seed mix.

Heat the avocado oil. Cook the chicken until golden brown and cooked within.

Divide the asparagus onto four serving plates, place a chicken on each, and garnish with the chili flakes. Serve warm.

Nutrition:

Calories: 451 kcal | Fat: 18.5 g | Carbs: 5.9 g | Fiber: 12.9 g | Protein: 19.5 g.

Part 2

NUTTY TEXTURED PORRIDGE

Prep time: 15 min

Cook time: 35 min

Servings: 05

Ingredients

½ cup pecans

½ cup walnuts

¼ cup sunflower seeds

¼ cup chia seeds

¼ cup unsweetened coconut flakes

4 cups unsweetened almond milk

½ tsp. ground cinnamon

¼ tsp. ground ginger

1 tsp. stevia powder

1 tbsp. butter.

Directions

1. In a food processor, place the pecans, walnuts and sunflower seeds and pulse until a crumbly mixture is formed.

2. In a large pan, add the nuts mixture, chia seeds, coconut flakes, almond milk, spices and stevia powder over medium heat and bring to a gentle simmer, stirring frequently.

3. Select heat to low and simmer for about 20-30 minutes, stirring frequently.

4. Remove from the heat and serve hot with the topping of butter.

Nutrition

Calories 269 kcal | Carbs: 8.6g | Protein: 7g.

PEAR & PEANUT BUTTER SMOOTHIE

Prep time: 10 min

Cook time: 0 min

Servings: 01

Ingredients

1 pear, peeled, cored and chopped

¾ cup unsweetened almond milk

½ tbsp. smooth peanut butter

½ tsp. fresh ginger, grated

¼ tsp. ground cinnamon

A handful of ice.

Directions

1. In a high-speed blender, combine all of the ingredients.

2. Blend until smooth, then transfer into a tall glasse filled with ice.

3. Top with pear and cinnamon crisps to serve (optional).

Nutrition

Calories 163 kcal | Fat: 5.5g | Carbs: 2g | Protein: 3.1g.

CHOCOLATE CHIA PUDDING

Prep time: 1 h 5 min

Cook time: 0 min

Servings: 04

Ingredients

½ cup black chia seeds

2 tbsp. unsweetened cocoa powder

4 tbsp. stevia

2 cups unsweetened almond milk

2 tsp. vanilla extract.

For Topping (optional)

Coconut yogurt

Seasonal fruit, sliced

Directions

1. In a large mixing bowl, combine chia seeds, sifted cocoa powder, and stevia. Stir well to remove any lumps.

2. Then add in the almond milk and vanilla extract and whisk until well combined.

3. Cover and refrigerate overnight (or for at least 1 hour).

4. Dish up the chocolate chia pudding right before serving. Add coconut yogurt and seasonal fruit. Enjoy!

Nutrition

Calories 335 kcal | Fat: 26.9g | Carbs: 15g | Protein: 8.2g.

KETO MUFFINS

Prep time: 10 min
Cook time: 23 min
Servings: 06

Ingredients

2 cups almond flour

½ cup powdered Swerve

3 scoops turmeric tonic

1½ tsp. organic baking powder

3 organic eggs

1 cup mayonnaise

½ tsp. organic vanilla extract.

Directions

1. Ready the oven to 350°F. Line a 12 cups muffin tin with paper liners.

2. In a large bowl, add the flour, Swerve, turmeric tonic and baking powder and mix well.

3. Add the eggs, mayonnaise and vanilla extract and beat until well combined. Place the mixture into the prepared muffin cups evenly. Bake for about 20-23 minutes.

4. Pull out the muffin tin. Position onto the wire rack to cool for 8 minutes.

5. Carefully invert the muffins onto the wire rack to cool completely before serving.

Nutrition

Calories 489 | Carbs: 9.5g | Protein: 10.8g.

BLUEBERRY WAFFLES

Prep time: 11 min

Cook time: 17 min

Servings: 09

Ingredients

8 eggs

5 oz. melted butter

1 tsp. vanilla extract

2 tsp. baking powder

⅓ cup coconut flour.

Topping:

3 oz. butter

1 oz. fresh blueberries.

Directions

1. Start by mixing the butter and eggs first until you get a smooth batter. Put in the remaining ingredients except those that you will be using as topping.

2. Heat your waffle iron to medium temperature and start pouring in the batter for cooking.

3. In a separate bowl, mix the butter and blueberries using a hand mixer. Use this to top off your freshly cooked waffles.

Nutrition

Calories 575 kcal | Fat 56g | Carbs: 15g | Fiber 5g | Protein: 36g.

KETO PANCAKES

Prep time: 5 min
Cook time: 15 min
Servings: 4-6

Ingredients

½ cup almond flour

4 oz. cream cheese, softened

4 large organic eggs

1 tsp. lemon zest

Butter, for frying and serving.

Directions

1. In a medium bowl, whisk together almond flour, cream cheese, eggs, and lemon zest until smooth.

2. In a nonstick skillet over medium-low heat, melt 1 tablespoon butter. Pour in about 3 tablespoons batter and cook until golden, 2 minutes.

3. Flip and cook 2 minutes more. Transfer to a plate and repeat with remaining batter.

4. You can serve it topped with butter and fresh berries. Enjoy!

Nutrition

Calories 110 kcal | Fat: 3.5g | Carbs: 2g | Protein: 4g.

JALAPENO POPPER EGG CUPS

Ingredients

5 large eggs

¾ tsp. salt

¼ tsp. black pepper

½ tsp. onion powder

½ tsp. garlic powder

½ cup Cheddar cheese, grated

⅓ cup cream cheese, softened

3-4 Jalapeno peppers, de-seeded and chopped

⅓ cup bacon, cooked crumbled.

Directions

1. Preheat the oven to 400°F and grease muffin tray with cooking spray. Set aside.

2. In a medium mixing bowl, whisk together eggs, onion powder, garlic powder, cream cheese, salt and pepper.

3. Stir in Cheddar cheese, chopped jalapeno peppers, and crumbled bacon. Mix until well combined.

4. Divide the mixture evenly into 6 muffin cups, filling each about 2/3 full.

5. Bake for about 12-15 minutes.

6. Serve hot.

Nutrition

Calories 120 kcal | Fat: 4g | Carbs: 1.4g | Protein: 5g.

SAVORY CHEDDAR OMELET

Prep time: 10 min
Cook time: 5 min
Servings: 04

Ingredients

4 large eggs

2 oz. cheddar cheese, shredded

8 olives, pitted

2 tbsp. butter

2 tbsp. olive oil

1 tsp. herb de Provence

½ tsp. salt.

Directions

1. Whisk eggs in a bowl with salt, olives, herb de Provence, and olive oil.

2. Melt butter in a large pan over medium heat.

3. Pour egg mixture into the hot pan and spread evenly.

4. Cover and cook for 3 minutes or until omelet lightly golden brown.

5. Flip omelet to the other side and cook for 2 minutes more.

6. Serve and enjoy!

Nutrition

Calories 251 kcal | Fat: 22g | Carbs 1.1g.

SPINACH & FETA BREAKFAST WRAPS

Prep time: 13 min

Cook time: 6 min

Servings: 02

Ingredients

1 tsp. olive oil

½ cup fresh baby spinach leaves

1 tbsp. fresh basil

4 egg whites, beaten

½ tsp. salt

¼ tsp. freshly ground black pepper

¼ cup crumbled low-fat feta cheese

2 (8-inch) whole-wheat tortillas.

Directions

1. Heat up olive oil on medium heat. Sauté spinach and basil to the pan for about 2 minutes.

2. Add the egg whites to the pan, season with the salt and pepper, and sauté, often stirring, for about 2 minutes more, or until the egg whites are firm.

3. Remove from the heat and sprinkle with the feta cheese.

4. Warm up tortillas in the microwave for 20 to 30 seconds. Divide the eggs between the tortillas and wrap up burrito-style.

Nutrition

Calories 224 kcal | Fat: 10.4g | Carbs: 4.5g | Protein: 10.6g.

AVOCADO TOASTS WITH 3 TOPPINGS

Prep time: 20 min

Cook time: 45 min

Servings: 03

Ingredients

Keto Seed Crackers:

1½ tbsp. almond flour

1½ tbsp. unsalted sunflower seeds

1½ tbsp. unsalted pumpkin seeds

1½ tbsp. flaxseed or chia seeds

1½ tbsp. sesame seeds

½ tbsp. ground psyllium husk powder

½ tsp. salt

1¼ tbsp. melted coconut oil

½ cup. boiling water.

Directions

Keto Seed Crackers:

1. Preheat the oven to 300°F.

2. Mix all dry ingredients in a bowl. Add boiling water and oil. Mix together well.

3. Keep working the dough until it forms a ball and has a gel-like consistency.

4. Place the dough on a baking sheet lined with parchment paper. Add another paper on top and use a rolling pin to flatten the dough evenly.

5. Remove the upper paper and bake on the lower rack for about 40-45 minutes, check occasionally. Seeds are heat sensitive so pay close attention towards the end.

6. Turn off the oven and leave the crackers to dry in the oven. Once dried and cool, break into 9 equal pieces and spread a generous amount of butter on top.

Toppings:

3 ripe avocados

3 lime3 (or lemon3)

Black pepper and sea salt, to taste

Fresh chili pepper, to taste

3 softly boiled or poached eggs

3 handfuls Romaine lettuce

3 pinches of parsley

6 fin slices of smoked (wild) salmon

3 handfuls mixed lettuce

3 pinches of dill.

Avocado Toasts:

7. Slice avocados lengthwise. Remove the seeds and the skin. Mash or slice avocados. Season with lime or lemon juice, black pepper and sea salt.

8. Top all the seed crackers with avocado.

9. Version 1: top 3 crackers with finely sliced chili pepper (seeds removed).

10. Version 2: top other 3 crackers with a softly boiled or poached eggs, finely chopped parsley and shredded Romaine lettuce.

11. Version 3: top last 3 crackers with smoked salmon, dill and mixed young lettuce leaves.

12. Enjoy!

Nutrition

Calories 224 kcal | Fat: 10.4g | Carbs: 4.5g | Protein: 10.6g.

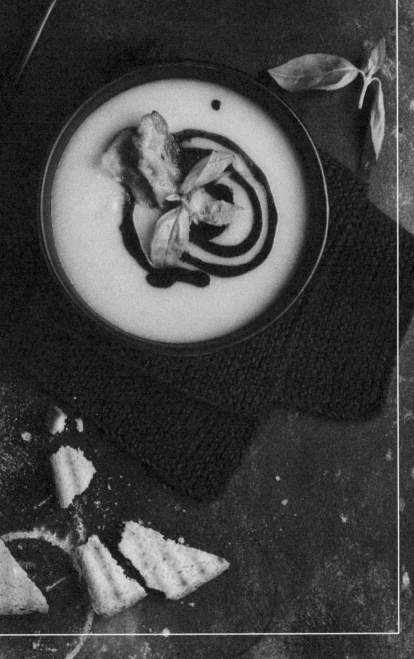

EASY SUMMER GAZPACHO

Ingredients

4 medium tomatoes chopped

1 English cucumber, peeled and chopped

¼ medium red onion, chopped

⅓ cup fresh parsley, chopped

12 fresh basil leaves

1 lemon juice

1 tbsp. extra-virgin olive oil

Salt and black pepper, to taste

½ cup grape tomatoes, quartered.

Directions

1. In a high-speed blender, combine all of the ingredients (except grape tomatoes), leaving apart ¼ of chopped cucumber, ¼ of chopped onion, ¼ of chopped parsley and 4 basil leaves.

2. Blend until smooth and creamy or about 2 minutes,

3. Then transfer into a large container, add in remaining chopped vegetables, cover and chill for 1 hour.

4. When ready to serve, divide the soup among 6 bowls and garnish with remaining herbs

Nutrition

Calories 92 kcal | Fat: 1.5g | Carbs: 10g | Protein: 2.3g.

FRESH AVOCADO SOUP

Prep time: 5 min

Cook time: 10 min

Servings: 02

Ingredients

1 ripe avocado

2 romaine lettuce leaves

1 cup coconut milk, chilled

1 tbsp. lime juice

20 fresh mint leaves.

Directions

1. Mix all your ingredients thoroughly in a blender.

2. Chill in the fridge for 5-10 minutes before serving.

Nutrition

Calories 280 kcal | Fat: 26g | Carbs: 2.6g | Protein: 4g

COLD ITALIAN CUCUMBER SOUP

Prep time: 2h 10min

Cook time: 0 min

Servings: 04

Ingredients

3 cucumbers, chopped

2 ripe avocados, peeled and pitted

2 spring onions, chopped

2 garlic cloves, minced

5 fresh basil leaves

2 tbsp. fresh parsley, chopped

2 cups vegetable stock

3 tbsp. lime juice

¼ cup extra virgin olive oil

Salt and black pepper, to taste.

Directions

1. In a high-speed blender combine chopped cucumbers, vegetable stock, avocado halves, lime juice, chopped onions, minced garlic cloves, basil leaves, and chopped parsley.

2. Process for 2-3 minutes, until smooth and creamy.

3. Transfer the soup into a container, cover and refrigerate for at least 2 hours before serving.

4. When ready to serve, pour the creamy chilled soup into 2 serving plates.

5. Top with the extra virgin olive oil, cucumber slices, basil leaves, dried tomatoes, and mozzarella halves.

6. Season with salt and pepper. Enjoy!

Nutrition

Calories 317 kcal | Fat: 25g | Carbs: 4.7g | Protein: 6g.

For Topping

3 tbsp. extra virgin olive oil

1 cucumber, thinly sliced

4 fresh basil leaves

4 dried tomatoes

8 little mozzarellas, halved

TOMATO SOUP & GRILLED CHEESE SANDWICHES

Prep time: 18 min

Cook time: 40 min

Servings: 04

Ingredients

3 tbsp. unsalted butter

1 tbsp. almond oil

1 (7 oz.) cans crushed tomatoes

2 medium white onions

1½ cups water

Salt and black pepper, to taste

1 tsp. dried basil

8 low-carb bread slices

1 cup Gruyere cheese

½ cup grated Monterey Jack cheese

Directions

1. Cook 2 tablespoons of butter in a pot and mix in the tomatoes, onions, and water.

2. Season with salt, black pepper, basil, and bring the mixture to a boil.

3. Reduce the heat immediately and simmer for 30 minutes or until the liquid reduces by a third.

4. Meanwhile, melt a ¼ tablespoon of butter in a non-stick skillet over medium heat and lay in a bread slice.

5. Add a quarter each of both cheese on top and cover with another bread slice.

6. Once the cheese starts melting and beneath the bread is golden brown, about 1 minute, flip the sandwich.

7. Cook further for 1 more minute or until the other side of the bread is golden brown too.

8. Remove the sandwich to a plate and make three more in the same manner.

9. Afterwards, diagonally slice each sandwich in half.

1 tbsp. chopped fresh basil for garnish.

10. Dish the tomato soup into serving bowls when ready, garnish with the basil leaves, and serve warm with the sandwiches.

Nutrition

Calories 285 kcal | Fat: 25.2g | Carbs: 13g | Protein: 12g.

CREAMY TAHINI ZOODLE SOUP

Prep time: 15min

Cook time: 14 min

Servings: 04

Ingredients

2 tbsp. coconut oil

2 tbsp. butter

½ medium onion, chopped

½ cup sliced cremini mushrooms

1 garlic clove, minced

4 cups vegetable broth

4 tbsp. coconut aminos

2 tbsp. erythritol

2 tbsp. tahini

4 tbsp. heavy cream

Directions

1. Warm up coconut oil and butter in a pot.

2. Stir-fry the onion, and mushrooms for 5 minutes or until softened.

3. Mix in the garlic and cook for 30 seconds or until fragrant.

4. Add the vegetable broth, coconut aminos, erythritol, tahini, heavy cream, and stir well. Boil the mix then, simmer for 5 minutes.

5. Mix in the zucchinis and cook for 3 minutes or until the zucchinis are tender.

6. Drizzle with the sesame oil, scallions, and sesame seeds.

Nutrition

4 zucchinis, spiralized.

Calories 347 kcal | Fat: 36g | Carbs: 6.5g | Protein: 11g.

For Topping

1 tbsp. toasted sesame oil

1 tbsp. chopped fresh scallions

1 tbsp. toasted sesame seeds.

GREEK EGG LEMON CHICKEN SOUP

Ingredients

4 cups of water

¾ lb. cauli

1 lb. boneless chicken thighs

⅓ lb. butter

4 eggs

1 lemon

2 tbsps. fresh parsley

1 bay leaf

2 chicken bouillon cubes

Salt and pepper.

Directions

1. Slice your chicken thinly and then place it in a saucepan while adding cold water and the cubes and bay leaf. Let the meat simmer for 10 mins before removing it and the bay leaf.

2. Grate your cauli and place it in a saucepan. Add butter and boil for a few minutes.

3. Beat your eggs and lemon juice in a bowl, while seasoning it.

4. Reduce the heat a bit and add the eggs, stirring continuously. Let simmer but don't boil.

5. Return in the chicken.

Nutrition

Calories 582 kcal | Fat: 49g | Carbs: 7.1g | Protein: 31g.

CAULIFLOWER RICE & CHICKEN SOUP

Prep time: 10 min
Cook time: 1 h
Servings: 05

Ingredients

2½ lb. chicken breasts

8 tbsp. butter

¼ cup celery, chopped

½ cup onion, chopped

4 cloves garlic, minced

2 (12-oz) packages steamed cauliflower rice

1 tbsp. parsley

2 tsp. poultry seasoning

½ cup carrot, grated

¾ tsp. rosemary

Salt and pepper

4 oz. cream cheese

4¾ cup chicken broth.

Directions

1. Put shredded chicken breasts into a saucepan and pour in the chicken broth. Add salt and pepper. Cook for 1 hour.

2. In another pot, melt the butter. Add the onion, garlic, and celery. Sauté until the mix is translucent. Add the rice cauliflower, rosemary, and carrot. Mix and cook for 7 minutes.

3. Mix chicken breasts and broth to the cauliflower mix. Put the lid on and simmer for 15 minutes.

Nutrition

Calories 415 kcal | Fat: 30g | Carbs: 9.8g | Protein: 27g

ASPARAGUS PUREE SOUP

Prep time: 15min

Cook time: 40 min

Servings: 04

Ingredients

2 tbsp. butter

1 garlic clove, minced

2 lb. asparagus, ends trimmed, cut into 1" pieces

2 cup low-sodium chicken broth

½ cup heavy cream

Salt and black pepper, to taste.

For Garnish

4 tbsp. heavy cream

4 tbsp. fresh chives, chopped

4 tbsp. fresh dill, chopped.

Directions

1. In a heavy pot over medium heat, melt butter. Add garlic and sauté for 1 minute.

2. Add asparagus and cook for about 5 minutes, until golden.

3. Add broth and simmer, covered for 10 to 15 minutes, until asparagus is tender but still green.

4. Puree the soup with an immersion blender. Then stir in heavy cream and warm over low heat. Season with salt and pepper to taste.

5. Dish up the soup, garnish with a spoon of heavy cream, fresh chives, and fresh dill. Serve hot.

Nutrition

Calories 246 kcal | Fat: 27g | Carbs: 5.9g | Protein: 10g.

CREAMY CHICKEN POT PIE SOUP

Prep time: 20 min

Cook time: 35 min

Servings: 06

Ingredients

2 tbsp. extra-virgin olive oil, divided

1 lb. skinless chicken breast

1 cup mushrooms, quartered

2 celery stalks, chopped

1 onion, chopped

1 tbsp. garlic, minced

5 cups low-sodium chicken broth

1 cup green beans, chopped

¼ cup cream cheese

1 cup heavy whipping cream

1 tbsp. fresh thyme, chopped.

Directions

1. Cook olive oil in a stockpot over medium-high heat until shimmering.

2. Add the chicken chunks to the pot and sauté for 10 minutes or until well browned.

3. Transfer the chicken to a plate. Set aside until ready to use.

4. Heat the remaining olive oil in the stockpot over medium-high heat.

5. Add the mushrooms, celery, onion, and garlic to the pot and sauté for 6 minutes or until fork-tender.

6. Pour the chicken broth over, then add the cooked chicken chunks to the pot. Stir to mix well and boil the soup. Adjust the heat to low. Simmer the for 15 minutes.

7. Mix in the green beans, cream cheese, cream, thyme, salt, and black pepper, then simmer for 3 more minutes. Serve Hot

Nutrition

Calories 338 kcal | Fat: 26.1g | Carbs: 24g | Protein: 28g.

CHUNKY PORK SOUP

Prep time: 25 min

Cook time: 30 min

Servings: 02

Ingredients

1 tbsp. olive oil

1 bell pepper, deveined and chopped

2 garlic cloves, pressed

½ cup scallions, chopped

½-pound ground pork (84% lean)

1 cup beef bone broth

1 cup of water

½ tsp. crushed red pepper flakes

1 bay laurel

1 tsp. fish sauce

2 cups mustard greens, torn into pieces

1 tbsp. fresh parsley, chopped.

Directions

1. Coat, once hot, sauté the pepper, garlic, and scallions until tender or about 3 minutes.

2. After that, stir in the ground pork and cook for 5 minutes more or until well browned, stirring periodically.

3. Add in the beef bone broth, water, red pepper, salt, black pepper, and bay laurel. Reduce the temperature to simmer and cook, covered, for 10 minutes. Afterward, stir in the fish sauce and mustard greens.

4. Remove from the heat; let it stand until the greens are wilted.

5. Ladle into individual bowls and serve garnished with fresh parsley.

Nutrition

Calories 344 kcal | Fat: 25.2g | Carbs: 12.1g | Protein: 23.1g.

CABBAGE SOUP WITH BEEF

Prep time: 15 min

Cook time: 20 min

Servings: 04

Ingredients

2 tbsp. olive oil

1 medium onion, chopped

1-pound fillet steak, cut into pieces

½ stalk celery, chopped

1 carrot, peeled and diced

½ head small green cabbage

2 cloves garlic, minced

4 cups beef broth

2 tbsp. fresh parsley, chopped

1 tsp. thyme, dried

1 tsp. rosemary, dried

1 tsp. garlic powder.

Directions

1. Heat oil in a pot (use medium heat). Add the beef and cook until it is browned. Put the onion into the pot and boil for 3-4 minutes.

2. Add the celery and carrot. Stir well and cook for about 3-4 minutes. Add the cabbage and boil until it starts softening. Add garlic and simmer for about 1 minute.

3. Pour the broth into the pot. Add the parsley and garlic powder. Mix thoroughly and reduce heat to medium-low.

4. Cook for 10-15 minutes.

Nutrition

Calories 177 kcal | Fat: 11g | Carbs: 3g | Protein: 12g.

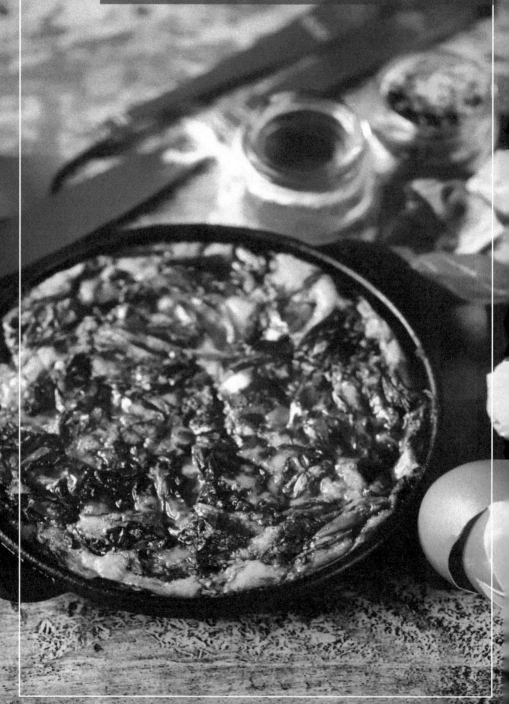

CITRUS EGG SALAD

Prep time: 10 min

Cook time: 20 min

Servings: 03

Ingredients

6 eggs

1 tsp. Dijon mustard

2 tbsp. of mayo

1 tsp. of lemon juice.

Directions

1. Place the eggs gently in a medium saucepan.
2. Add cold water until your eggs are covered by an inch.
3. Bring to a boil.
4. You should do this for ten minutes. Remove from your heat and cool. Peel your eggs under running water that is cold.
5. Put your eggs in a food processor. Pulse until they are chopped.
6. Stir in condiments and juice.

Nutrition

Calories 22 kcal | Fat: 19g | Carbs: 8g | Protein: 13g.

TOMATO & MOZZA SALAD

Prep time: 15 min

Cook time: 10 min

Servings: 08

Ingredients

4 cups cherry tomatoes

1½ lb. mozzarella cheese

¼ cup fresh basil leaves

¼ cup olive oil

2 tbsp. fresh lemon juice

1 tsp. fresh oregano

1 tsp. fresh parsley

3 drops liquid stevia.

Directions

1. In a salad bowl, mix together tomatoes, mozzarella, and basil.
2. In a small bowl, add remaining ingredients and beat until well combined.
3. Place dressing over salad and toss to coat well.
4. Serve immediately.

Nutrition

Calories 87 kcal | Fat: 7.5g | Carbs: 5.2g | Protein: 2.4g.

SHRIMP LETTUCE WRAPS WITH BUFFALO SAUCE

Prep time: 15 min
Cook time: 20 min
Servings: 04

Ingredients

1 egg, beaten

3 tbsp. butter

16 oz. shrimp, peeled, deveined, with tails removed

¾ cup almond flour

¼ cup hot sauce (like Frank's)

1 tsp. extra-virgin olive oil

1 head romaine lettuce, leaves parted, for serving

½ red onion, chopped

Celery, finely sliced

½ blue cheese, cut into pieces.

Directions

1. To make the Buffalo sauce, melt the butter in a saucepan, add the garlic and cook this mixture for 1 minute. Pour hot sauce into the saucepan and whisk to combine. Set aside.

2. In one bowl, crack one egg, add salt and pepper and mix. In another bowl, put the almond flour, add salt and pepper and also combine. Dip each shrimp into the egg mixture first and then into the almond one.

3. Take a large frying pan. Heat the oil and cook your shrimp for about 2 minutes per side. Add Buffalo sauce

4. Serve in lettuce leaves. Top your shrimp with red onion, blue cheese, and celery.

Nutrition

Calories 213 kcal | Fat: 54g | Carbs: 8g | Protein: 33g.

CREAMY KETO EGG SALAD

Prep time: 5 min

Cook time: 15 min

Servings: 04

Ingredients

8 large eggs, boiled

1/2 cup low carb mayonnaise

1 tbsp. chives, finely chopped

1 tsp. lemon juice

2 tsp. Dijon mustard

½ tsp. salt

¼ tsp. freshly ground black pepper

A pinch of paprika.

Directions

1. Peel and dice the eggs.
2. In a mixing bowl combine all of the ingredients and stir gently.
3. Adjust salt and pepper to taste and serve.

Nutrition

Calories 413 kcal | Fat: 10g | Carbs: 2g | Protein: 12g.

SMOKED SALMON FILLED AVOCADOS

Prep time: 13 min
Cook time: 5 min
Servings: 02

Ingredients

1 medium avocado

3 oz. smoked salmon

4 tbsp. sour cream

1 tbsp. lemon juice

Pepper and salt, to taste.

Directions

1. Cut the avocado into two and discard the pit.

2. Place the same amounts of sour cream in the hollow parts of the avocado. Include smoked salmon on top.

3. Season with pepper and salt, squeeze lemon juice over the top.

Nutrition

Calories 517 kcal | Fats: 42.6g | Carbs: 5.9g | Protein: 20.6g.

MUSHROOM OMELET

Ingredients

3 medium eggs

1 oz. cheese, shredded

1 oz. butter used for frying

¼ yellow onion, chopped

4 large mushrooms, sliced

Your favorite vegetables (optional).

Directions

1. Scourge eggs in a bowl. Add some salt and pepper to taste.

2. Cook butter in a pan using low heat. Put in the mushroom and onion, cooking the two until you get that amazing smell.

3. Pour the egg mix into the pan and allow it to cook on medium heat. Allow the bottom part to cook before sprinkling the cheese on top of the still-raw portion of the egg.

4. Carefully pry the edges of the omelet and fold it in half. Allow it to cook for a few more seconds before removing the pan from the heat and sliding it directly onto your plate.

Nutrition

Calories 520 kcal | Fat: 27g | Carbs: 5g | Protein: 26g.

AVOCADO TACO

Prep time: 10 min
Cook time: 15 min
Servings: 06

Ingredients

1-pound ground beef

3 avocados, halved

1 tbsp. Chili powder

½ tsp. salt

¾ tsp. cumin

½ tsp. oregano, dried

¼ tsp. garlic powder

¼ tsp. onion powder

8 tbsp. tomato sauce

1 cup Cheddar cheese, shredded

¼ cup cherry tomatoes, sliced

¼ cup lettuce, shredded

½ cup sour cream.

Directions

1. Pit halved avocados. Set aside.

2. Place the ground beef into a saucepan. Cook at medium heat until it is browned.

3. Add the seasoning and tomato sauce. Stir well and cook for about 4 minutes.

4. Load each avocado half with the beef.

5. Top with shredded cheese and lettuce, tomato slices, and sour cream.

Nutrition

Calories 278 kcal | Fat: 22g | Carbs: 14g | Protein: 18g.

KETO CAESAR SALAD

Ingredients

1½ cup mayonnaise

3 tbsp. apple cider vinegar/acv

1 tsp. Dijon mustard

4 anchovy filets

24 romaine heart leaves

4 oz. pork rinds, chopped

Parmesan (for garnish).

Directions

1. Place the mayo with ACV, mustard, and anchovies into a blender and process until smooth and dressing like.

2. Prepare romaine leaves and pour out dressing across them evenly. Top with pork rinds and enjoy.

Nutrition

Calories 400 kcal | Fat: 25g | Carbs: 9g | Protein: 33g.

CHICKEN CLUB LETTUCE WRAP

Prep time: 15 min

Cook time: 15 min

Servings: 01

Ingredients

1 head of iceberg lettuce with the core and outer leaves removed

1 tbsp. of mayonnaise

6 slices or organic chicken or turkey breast

2 cooked strips of bacon

2 slices tomato

Directions

1. Line your working surface with a large slice of parchment paper. Layer 6-8 large leaves of lettuce in the center of the paper to make a base of around 9-10 inches. Spread the mayo in the center and lay with chicken or turkey, bacon, and tomato.

2. Starting with the end closest to you, roll the wrap like a jelly roll with the parchment paper as your guide. Keep it tight and halfway through, roll tuck in the ends of the wrap.

3. When it is completely wrapped, roll the rest of the parchment paper around it, and use a knife to cut it in half.

Nutrition

Calories 207 kcal | Carbs: 6g | Protein: 12g | Fat: 15g.

SCALLOPS IN GARLIC SAUCE

Prep time: 15 min

Cook time: 13 min

Servings: 04

Ingredients

1¼ lb. fresh sea scallops

4 tbsp. butter, divided

5 garlic cloves, chopped

¼ cup homemade chicken broth

1 cup heavy cream

1 tbsp. fresh lemon juice

2 tbsp. fresh parsley.

Directions

1. Sprinkle the scallops evenly with salt and black pepper.

2. Melt 2 tablespoons of butter in a large pan over medium-high heat and cook the scallops for about 2–3 minutes per side.

3. Flip the scallops and cook for about 2 more minutes.

4. With a slotted spoon, transfer the scallops onto a plate.

5. Now, melt the remaining butter in the same pan over medium heat and sauté the garlic for about 1 minute.

6. Pour the broth and bring to a gentle boil. Cook for about 2 minutes. Stir in the cream and cook for about 1–2 minutes or until slightly thickened.

7. Stir in the cooked scallops and lemon juice and remove from heat. Garnish with fresh parsley and serve hot.

Nutrition

Calories 435 kcal | Fat: 33g | Carbs: 12.4g | Protein: 25g.

BUTTER TROUT WITH BOK CHOY

Prep time: 15 min

Cook time: 30 min

Servings: 06

Ingredients

½ tbsp. honey

1 tbsp. tamari

1 large garlic clove

¾ tsp. chili powder

1 filet (6 oz.) trout fish

2 heads baby bok choy

½ tsp. sesame oil

¼ tsp. hot pepper flakes.

Directions

1. Prep oven to 425°F and line a baking sheet with parchment paper.

2. Scourge honey, half the tamari, minced garlic and chili powder.

3. Arrange rainbow trout skin side down onto parchment paper and season. Use a brush to spread the honey garlic mixture onto the fish.

4. Toss bok choy to a large mixing bowl and drizzle with the remaining tamari and sesame oil. Situate bok choy to baking sheet and organize it around the rainbow trout. Bake for 12 to 15 minutes.

Nutrition

Calories 352 kcal | Fat: 37g | Carbs: 2g | Protein: 42.5g.

BUTTER CHICKEN

Prep time: 15 min

Cook time: 30 min

Servings: 05

Ingredients

3 tbsp. unsalted butter

1 medium yellow onion, chopped

2 garlic cloves, minced

1 tsp. fresh ginger, minced

1½ lb. grass-fed chicken breasts

2 tomatoes, chopped finely

1 tbsp. garam masala

1 tsp. red chili powder

1 tsp. ground cumin

1 cup heavy cream

2 tbsp. fresh cilantro.

Directions

1. Cook butter in a large wok over medium-high heat and sauté the onions for about 5–6 minutes. Add in ginger and garlic and sauté for about 1 minute. Add the tomatoes and cook for about 2–3 minutes, crushing with the back of spoon.

2. Stir in the chicken spices, salt, and black pepper, and cook for about 6–8 minutes or until desired doneness of the chicken.

3. Drizzle the heavy cream and cook for about 8–10 more minutes, stirring occasionally. Garnish with fresh cilantro and serve hot.

Nutrition

Calories 507 kcal | Fat: 33g | Carbs: 14g | Protein: 41g.

BACON ROASTED CHICKEN WITH PAN GRAVY

Prep time: 8 min

Cook time: 1h 5 min

Servings: 08

Ingredients

3 lb. whole chicken, gutted

4 sprigs fresh thyme

1 medium lemon

10 strips bacon

Salt and pepper to taste

1 tbsp. grain mustard.

Directions

1. Oven preheats to 500°F.

2. Season chicken with salt and pepper, then lemon stuff, and thyme. Cover bacon with salt and pepper over bird skin, and season bacon.

3. Place the bird in a roasting saucepan and place it in the oven for 15 minutes. Reduce the temperature to 350°F and bake for 40-50 minutes.

4. Remove the bird and put it in foil.

5. Drizzle the juices into a pan and bring to a boil.

6. Add mustard, stir in, and slightly reduce to pan liquids. Then, use an immersion blender to blend sauce into the pan.

7. Serve with gravy on chicken.

Nutrition

Calories 376 | Fats: 29.8g | Carbs: 6.1g | Protein: 24.5g.

CHICKEN WITH MEDITERRANEAN SAUCE

Prep time: 4 min

Cook time: 16 min

Servings: 06

Ingredients

1 stick butter

½ pounds of chicken breasts

2 tsp. red wine vinegar

½ tbsp. olive oil

⅓ cup fresh Italian parsley, chopped

1 tbsp. green garlic

2 tbsp. red onions

Flaky sea salt and ground black pepper, to taste.

Directions

1. In a cast-iron skillet, heat the oil over a moderate flame. Sear the chicken for 10 to 12 minutes or until no longer pink. Season with salt and black pepper.

2. Add in the melted butter and continue to cook until heated through. Stir in the green garlic, onion, and Italian parsley; let it cook for 3 to 4 minutes more.

3. Mix in red wine vinegar and pull away from the heat.

Nutrition

Calories 411 kcal | Fat: 21g | Carbs: 19.7g | Protein: 36g.

TURKEY-PEPPER MIX

Prep time: 20 min

Cook time: 0 min

Servings: 01

Ingredients

1-pound turkey tenderloin

1 tsp. salt, divided

2 tbsp. extra-virgin olive oil

½ sweet onion, sliced

1 red bell pepper, cut into strips

1 yellow bell pepper, cut into strips

½ tsp. Italian seasoning

¼ tsp. ground black pepper

2 tsp. red wine vinegar

1 (14-ounces) can crush tomatoes.

Directions

1. Sprinkle ½ teaspoon salt on your turkey. Pour 1 tablespoon oil into the pan and heat it. Add the turkey steaks and cook for 1-3 minutes per side. Set aside.

2. Put the onion, bell peppers, and the remaining salt to the pan and cook for 7 minutes, stirring all the time. Sprinkle with Italian seasoning and add black pepper. Cook for 30 seconds. Add the tomatoes and vinegar and fry the mix for about 20 seconds.

3. Return the turkey to the pan and pour the sauce over it. Simmer for 2-3 minutes. Top with chopped parsley and basil.

Nutrition

Calories 230 kcal | Fat: 8g | Carbs: 6.8g | Protein: 30g.

CHICKEN PAN WITH VEGGIES & PESTO

Ingredients

2 tbsp. olive oil

1-pound chicken thighs

¾ cup oil-packed sun-dried tomatoes

1-pound asparagus ends

¼ cup basil pesto

1 cup cherry tomatoes, red and yellow.

Directions

1. Cook olive oil in a frying pan over medium-high heat.

2. Put salt on the chicken slices and the put into a skillet, add the sun-dried tomatoes and fry for 5-10 minutes. Remove the chicken slices and season with salt. Add asparagus to the skillet. Cook for additional 5-10 minutes.

3. Position the chicken back in the skillet, pour in the pesto and whisk. Fry for 1-2 minutes. Remove from the heat. Add the halved cherry tomatoes and pesto. Stir well and serve.

Nutrition

Calories 423 kcal | Fat: 32g | Carbs: 8.9g | Protein: 2g.

CHICKEN QUESADILLAS

Prep time: 10 min
Cook time: 15 min
Servings: 02

Ingredients

1½ cups Mozzarella cheese, shredded

1½ cups Cheddar cheese, shredded

1 cup chicken, cooked and shredded

1 bell pepper, sliced

¼ cup tomato, diced

⅛ cup green onion

1 tbsp. extra-virgin olive oil

Directions

1. Preheat the oven to 400°F. Use parchment paper to cover a pizza pan.

2. Combine your cheeses and bake the cheese shell for about 5 minutes.

3. Put the chicken on one half of the cheese shell. Add peppers, tomatoes, green onion and fold your shell in half over the fillings.

4. Return your folded cheese shell to the oven again for 4-5 minutes.

Nutrition

Calories 244 kcal | Fat: 40.5g | Carbs: 6.1g. | Protein: 52.7g.

CREAMY GARLIC CHICKEN

Prep time: 5 min

Cook time: 15 min

Servings: 04

Ingredients

4 chicken breasts

1 tsp. garlic powder

1 tsp. paprika

2 tbsp. butter

1 tsp. salt

1 cup heavy cream

½ cup sun-dried tomatoes

2 cloves garlic

1 cup spinach.

Directions

1. Blend the paprika, garlic powder, and salt and sprinkle over both sides of the chicken.

2. Melt the butter in a frying pan (choose medium heat). Add the chicken breast and fry for 5 minutes each side. Set aside.

3. Add the heavy cream, sun-dried tomatoes, and garlic to the pan and whisk well to combine. Cook for 2 minutes. Add spinach and sauté for an additional 3 minutes.

4. Return the chicken to the pan and cover with the sauce

Nutrition

Calories 280 kcal | Fat: 26g | Carbs: 8g | Protein: 4g.

EASY ONE-PAN GROUND BEEF AND GREEN BEANS

Prep time: 13 min

Cook time: 6 min

Servings: 02

Ingredients

10 oz. (18-20) ground beef

9 oz. green beans

Pepper and salt, to taste

2 tbsp. sour cream

3½ oz. butter.

Directions

1. Rinse green beans, then trim the ends off each side.

2. Place half of the butter to a pan (that can fit the ground green beans and beef) over high heat.

3. Once hot, stir in the ground beef and season. Cook the beef until it's almost done.

4. Set heat on the pan to medium. Cook rest of butter and green beans to the pan for five minutes. Stir the ground beef and green beans rarely.

5. Season the green beans, with the pan drippings.

Nutrition

Calories 787.5 kcal | Fats: 71.75g | Carbs: 0.6g | Protein: 27.5g.

SHEET PAN BURGERS

Prep time: 12 min

Cook time: 17 min

Servings: 03

Ingredients

24 oz. ground beef

Sea salt & pepper, to taste

½ tsp. garlic powder

6 slices bacon, halved

1 med. onion, sliced into ¼ rounds

2 jalapeños, seeded & sliced

4 slices pepper jack cheese

¼ cup mayonnaise

1 tbsp. chili sauce

½ tsp. Worcestershire sauce

8 lg. leaves of Boston or butter lettuce

8 dill pickle chips.

Directions

1. Prep the oven to 425°F and line a baking sheet with non-stick foil.

2. Mix the salt, pepper, and garlic into the ground beef and form 4 patties out of it.

3. Line the burgers, bacon slices, jalapeño slices, and onion rounds onto the baking sheet and bake for about 18 minutes.

4. Garnish each patty with a piece of cheese and set the oven to boil.

5. Broil for 2 minutes, then remove the pan from the oven.

6. Serve one patty with 3 pieces of bacon, jalapeño slices, onion rounds, and desired amount of sauce with 2 pickle chips and 2 pieces of lettuce.

Nutrition

Calories 608 kcal | Fat: 46g | Carbs: 5g | Protein: 42g.

RICH AND EASY PORK RAGOUT

Prep time: 15 min

Cook time: 45 min

Servings: 04

Ingredients

1 tsp. lard, melted at room temperature

¾-pound pork butt

1 red bell pepper

1 poblano pepper

2 cloves garlic

½ cup leeks

½ tsp. mustard seeds

¼ tsp. ground allspice

¼ tsp. celery seeds

1 cup roasted vegetable broth

2 vine-ripe tomatoes, pureed.

Directions

1. Melt the lard in a stockpot over moderate heat. Once hot, cook the pork cubes for 4 to 6 minutes, occasionally stirring to ensure even cooking.

2. Then, stir in the vegetables and continue cooking until they are tender and fragrant. Add in the salt, black pepper, mustard seeds, allspice, celery seeds, roasted vegetable broth, and tomatoes.

3. Reduce the heat to simmer. Let it simmer for 30 minutes longer or until everything is heated through. Ladle into individual bowls and serve hot.

Nutrition

Calories 389 kcal | Fat 24.3g | Carbs: 5.4g | Protein: 22.7g.

MEXICAN CASSEROLE

Ingredients

1-pound lean ground beef

2 cups salsa

1 (16 oz.) can chili beans, drained

3 cups tortilla chips, crushed

2 cups sour cream

1 (2 oz.) can slice black olives, drained

½ cup chopped green onion

½ cup chopped fresh tomato

2 cups shredded Cheddar cheese.

Directions

1. Prep oven to 350°F.

2. In a big wok over medium heat, cook the meat so that it is no longer pink. Add the sauce, reduce the heat and simmer for 20 minutes or until the liquid is absorbed. Add beans and heat.

3. Sprinkle a 9x13 baking dish with oil spray. Pour the chopped tortillas into the pan and then place the meat mixture on it.

4. Pour sour cream over meat and sprinkle with olives, green onions, and tomatoes. Top with cheddar cheese.

5. Bake in preheated oven for 30 minutes or until hot and bubbly.

Nutrition

Calories 597 kcal | Fat: 43.7g | Carbs: 32.8g | Protein: 31.7g.

PULLED PORK, MINT & CHEESE

Prep time: 20 min
Cook time: 15 min
Servings: 02

Ingredients

1 tsp. lard, melted at room temperature

¾ pork Boston butt, sliced

2 garlic cloves, pressed

½ tsp. red pepper flakes, crushed

½ tsp. black peppercorns, freshly cracked

Sea salt, to taste

2 bell peppers, deveined and sliced

1 tbsp. fresh mint leave snipped

4 tbsp. cream cheese.

Directions

1. Melt the lard in a cast-iron skillet over a moderate flame. Once hot, brown the pork for 2 minutes per side until caramelized and crispy on the edges.

2. Reduce the temperature to medium-low and continue cooking another 4 minutes, turning over periodically. Shred the pork with two forks and return to the skillet.

3. Add the garlic, red pepper, black peppercorns, salt, and bell pepper and continue cooking for a further 2 minutes or until the peppers are just tender and fragrant.

4. Serve with fresh mint and a dollop of cream cheese. Enjoy!

Nutrition

Calories 370 kcal | Fat: 21.9g | Carbs: 16g | Protein: 34.9g.

PORK CHOP

Prep time: 10 min

Cook time: 30 min

Servings: 02

Ingredients

12 pork chops, boneless, thin cut

2 cups baby spinach

4 cloves of garlic

12 slices Provolone cheese.

Directions

1. Prep oven to a temperature of 350°F.

2. Pound the garlic cloves using a garlic press. The cloves should go through the press and into a small bowl.

3. Spread the garlic that you have made onto one side of the pork chops.

4. Flip half a dozen chops while making sure the garlic side is down. You should do this on a baking sheet that is rimmed.

5. Divide your spinach between the half dozen chops.

6. Fold cheese slices in half. Situate them on top of spinach.

7. Position the second pork chop on top of the first set, but this time make sure that the garlic side is up.

8. Bake for 20 minutes.

9. Cover each chop with another piece of cheese.

10. Bake another 15 minutes.

11. Your meat meter should be at 160°F when you check with a thermometer.

12. Serve hot and enjoy!

Nutrition

Calories 436 kcal | Fat: 25g | Carbs: 9.2g | Protein: 47g.

CAULIFLOWER CASSEROLE

Prep time: 15 min

Cook time: 35 min

Servings: 04

Ingredients

1 large head cauliflower

2 tbsp. butter

2 oz. cream cheese

1¼ cup sharp cheddar cheese

1 cup heavy cream

¼ cup scallion.

Directions

1. Preheat the oven to 350°F.

2. In a huge pan of boiling water, mix the cauliflower florets and cook for about 2 minutes.

3. Drain cauliflower and keep aside.

4. For cheese sauce: in a medium pan, add butter over medium-low heat and cook until just melted.

5. Add cream cheese, 1 cup of cheddar cheese, heavy cream, salt and black pepper and cook until melted and smooth, stirring continuously.

6. Pull away from heat and keep aside to cool slightly.

7. In a baking dish, place cauliflower florets, cheese sauce, and 3 tablespoons of scallion and stir to combine well.

8. Sprinkle with remaining cheddar cheese and scallion.

9. Bake for about 30 minutes.

10. Remove the casserole dish from oven and set aside for about 5-10 minutes before serving.

11. Cut into 4 equal-sized portions and serve.

Nutrition

Calories 365 kcal | Fat: 14g | Carbs: 5.6g | Protein: 12g.

RICOTTA & BEEF STUFFED ZUCCHINI

Prep time: 15 min

Cook time: 30 min

Servings: 04

Ingredients

4 medium zucchini

1/2 lb. ground beef

2 large eggs

¾ cup part-skim Ricotta cheese

½ cup Parmesan cheese, grated

1 garlic clove,, minced

1 tbsp. dried basil

1 tbsp. fresh parsley, chopped

¾ tsp. salt

¼ tsp. ground black pepper

Extra virgin olive oil for drizzling.

Directions

1. Preheat the oven to 450°F. Line a baking sheet with parchment paper.
2. Half zucchini lengthwise. Remove the pulp from the center with a teaspoon, keeping the skin intact.
3. In a large bowl combine finely chopped zucchini pulp with all of the other ingredients and mix well. Divide the mixture between 8 zucchini halves.
4. Arrange stuffed zucchini on baking sheet, sprinkle with a little salt and drizzle with olive oil. Bake for 25-30 minutes until zucchini is tender and filling is beginning to brown. Serve hot.

Nutrition

Calories 322 kcal | Fat 20g | Carbs: 8g | Protein: 14g.

SNACK & SIDE RECIPES

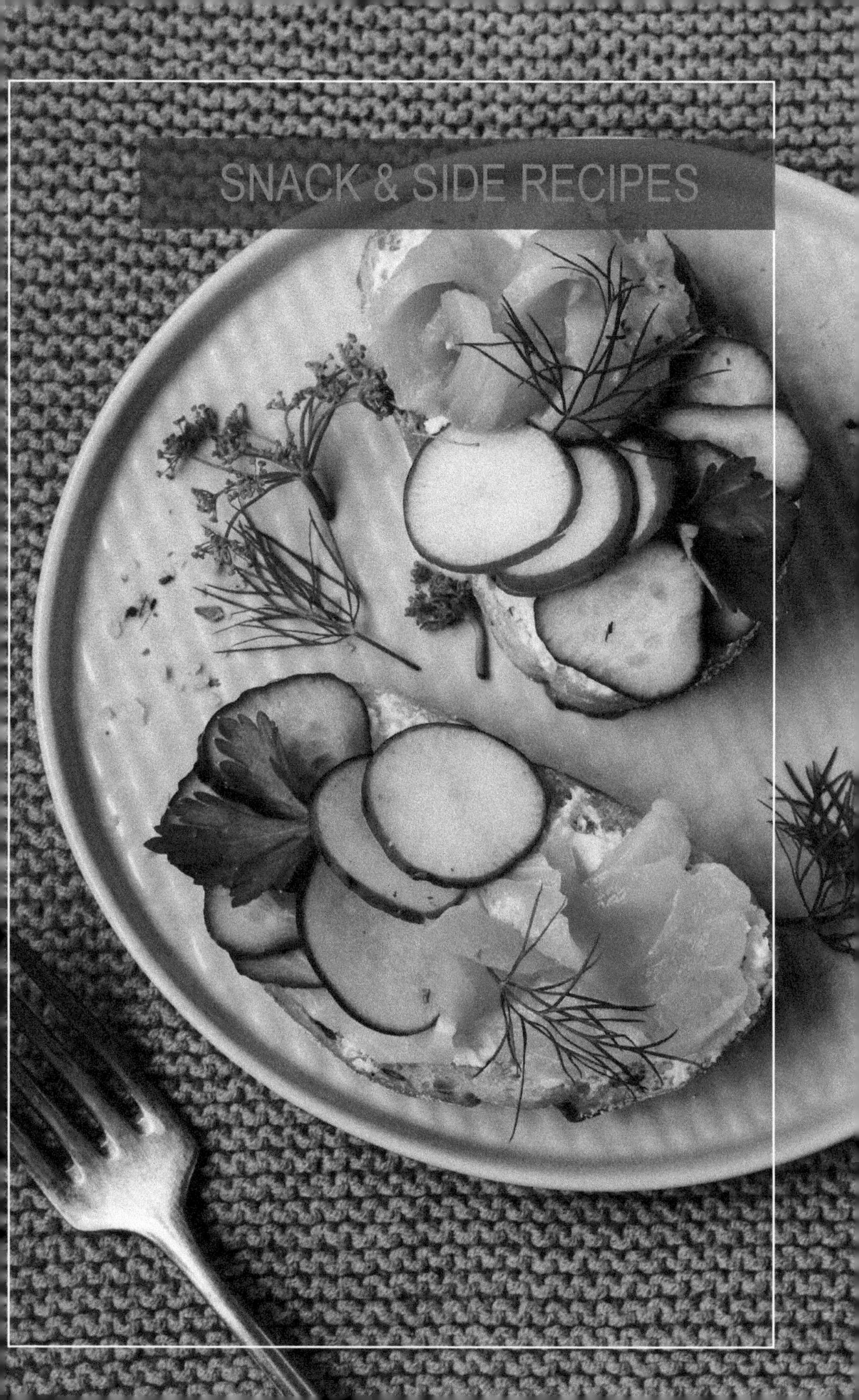

CAULIFLOWER BREADSTICKS

Prep time: 10 min

Cook time: 1h 35min

Servings: 04

Ingredients

4 eggs

4 cups of cauliflower riced

2 cups mozzarella cheese

4 cloves minced garlic

3 tsp. oregano.

Directions

1. Ready oven to 425°F. Line baking sheet by using parchment paper.

2. Situate cauliflower in a food processor or blender until finely chopped or when it resembles rice.

3. Put it in a covered bowl and microwave for just 10 minutes. Allow it to cool and if it's a little wet, make sure to drain it first before adding eggs, oregano, garlic, salt, pepper, and mozzarella. Mix them well.

4. Start separating the mixture into individual sticks – or really, just about any form you want.

5. Bake for 25 minutes. Pull out form the oven and sprinkle some more mozzarella on top while still hot. Put it back in the oven for just 5 minutes so that the cheese melts.

Nutrition

Calories 99 kcal | Fat: 19g | Carbs: 4g | Protein: 13g.

SPINACH IN CHEESE ENVELOPES

Prep time: 15 min

Cook time: 30 min

Servings: 08

Ingredients

3 cup cream cheese

1½ cup coconut flour

3 egg yolks

2 eggs

½ cup cheddar cheese

2 cups steamed spinach

¼ tsp. salt

½ tsp. pepper

¼ c. chopped onion.

Directions

1. Place cream cheese in a mixing bowl then whisks until soft and fluffy.

2. Add egg yolks to the mixing bowl then continue whisking until incorporated.

3. Stir in coconut flour to the cheese mixture then mix until becoming a soft dough.

4. Place the dough on a flat surface then roll until thin.

5. Cut the thin dough into 8 squares then keep.

6. Crash the eggs then place in a bowl. Season with salt, pepper, and grated cheese then mix well.

7. Add chopped spinach and onion to the egg mixture then stir until combined.

8. Put spinach filling on a square dough then fold until becoming an envelope.

9. Repeat with the remaining spinach filling and dough. Glue with water.

10. Preheat an Air Fryer to 425°F. Arrange the spinach envelopes in the Air Fryer then cook for 12 minutes or until lightly golden brown.

11. Remove from the Air Fryer then serve warm. Enjoy!

Nutrition

Calories 365 kcal | Fat: 34g | Protein: 10g.

MOZZARELLA CHEESE POCKETS

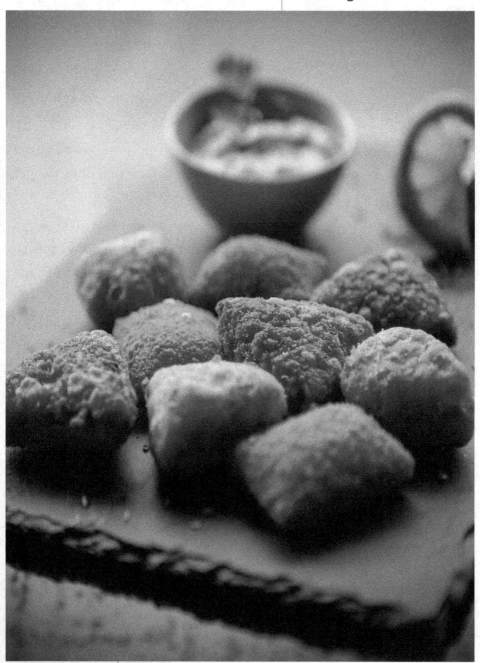

Ingredients

Directions

1 large egg

8 pcs. of mozzarella cheese sticks

1¾ cup mozzarella cheese

¾ cup almond flour

1 oz. cream cheese

½ cup of crushed pork rinds.

1. Start by grating the mozzarella cheese.

2. Scourge the almond flour, mozzarella, and the cream cheese. Microwave them for 3 seconds until you get that delicious gooey mixture.

3. Put in a large egg and mix the whole thing together. You should get a nice thick batch of dough.

4. Put the dough in between two wax papers and roll it around until you get a semi-rectangular shape

5. Cut them into smaller rectangle pieces and wrap them around the cheese sticks. Mold it depending on the shape you want.

6. Roll the stick onto crushed pork rinds. Bake for 20 to 25 minutes at 400°F.

Nutrition

Calories 272 kcal | Fat: 22g | Carbs: 11g | Protein: 17g.

CATFISH BITES

Prep time: 12 min

Cook time: 16 min

Servings: 06

Ingredients

1-pound catfish fillet

1 tsp. minced garlic

1 large egg

½ onion, diced

1 tbsp. butter, melted

1 tsp. turmeric

1 tsp. ground thyme

1 tsp. ground coriander

¼ tsp. ground nutmeg

1 tsp. flax seeds.

Directions

1. Cut the catfish fillet into 6 bites.
2. Sprinkle the fish bites with the minced garlic. Stir it.
3. Then add diced onion, turmeric, ground thyme, ground coriander, ground nutmeg, and flax seeds. Mix the catfish bites gently.
4. Prep air fryer to 360°F.
5. Spray the catfish bites with the melted butter. Then freeze them.
6. Put the catfish bites in the air fryer basket and cook for 16 minutes.
7. When the dish is cooked – chill it. Enjoy!

Nutrition

Calories 140 kcal | Protein: 13.1g | Fats: 8.7g | Carbs: 4.2g.

KETO EGGS & PORK CUPS

Prep time: 15 min

Cook time: 40 min

Servings: 06

Ingredients

Cooking spray, for pan

2 lb. ground pork

2 cloves garlic, minced

½ tsp. paprika

1 tbsp. freshly chopped thyme

½ tsp. ground cumin

1 tsp. salt

Freshly ground black pepper, to taste

2½ cup chopped fresh spinach

1 cup shredded white cheddar

12 eggs

1 tbsp. freshly chopped chives.

Directions

1. Preheat oven to 400°F.

2. In a large bowl, combine ground pork, garlic, paprika, thyme, cumin, salt and pepper.

3. Prep 12 cups muffin tin with cooking spray. Add a small handful of pork to each muffin tin well then press up the sides to create a cup.

4. Divide spinach and cheese evenly between cups. Crack an egg on top of each cup and season with salt and pepper. Bake until eggs are set, and pork is cooked through, about 25 minutes.

5. Garnish with chives and serve. Enjoy!

Nutrition

Calories 385 kcal | Fat: 39g | Carbs: 3g | Protein: 16g.

ZUCCHINI MUFFINS

Prep time: 15 min
Cook time: 15 min
Servings: 04

Ingredients

4 organic eggs

¼ cup unsalted butter, melted

¼ cup water

⅓ cup coconut flour

½ tsp. organic baking powder

¼ tsp. salt

1½ cups zucchini, grated

½ cup Parmesan cheese, shredded

1 tbsp. fresh oregano, minced

1 tbsp. fresh thyme, minced

¼ cup cheddar cheese, grated.

Directions

1. Preheat the oven to 400ºF.

2. Lightly, grease 8 muffin tins.

3. Add eggs, butter, and water in a mixing bowl and beat until well combined.

4. Add the flour, baking powder, and salt, and mix well.

5. Add remaining ingredients except for cheddar and mix until just combined.

6. Place the mixture into prepared muffin cups evenly.

7. Bake for approximately 13–15 minutes or until top of muffins become golden-brown.

8. Remove the muffin tin from oven and situate onto a wire rack for 10 minutes.

9. Carefully invert the muffins onto a platter and serve warm.

Nutrition

Calories 287 kcal | Fat: 23g | Carbs: 8.7g | Protein: 13.2g.

KETO GARLIC BREAD

Prep time: 5 min

Cook time: 30 min

Servings: 04

Ingredients

1 cup Mozzarella cheese, shredded

½ cup almond flour

2 tbsp. cream cheese

1 tbsp. garlic powder

1 tsp. baking powder

Salt, to taste

1 large egg

1 tbsp. butter, melted

1 clove garlic, minced

1 tbsp. freshly chopped parsley

1 tbsp. Parmesan cheese, freshly grated

Marinara, warmed, for serving.

Directions

1. Preheat oven to 400°F and line a large baking sheet with parchment paper.

2. In a medium, microwave-safe bowl, add mozzarella, almond flour, cream cheese, garlic powder, baking powder, and a large pinch of salt. Microwave on high until cheeses are melted, about 1 minute. Stir in egg. Shape dough into a baking sheet.

3. In a small bowl, mix melted butter with garlic, parsley, and Parmesan. Brush mixture over top of bread. Bake until golden, 15 to 17 minutes. Slice and serve with marinara sauce for dipping.

Nutrition

Calories 250 kcal | Fat: 20g | Carbs: 7g | Protein: 13g.

BRIE CHEESE FAT BOMBS

Prep time: 45 min
Cook time: 3 min
Servings: 06

Ingredients

2 oz. cream cheese, full fat

½ cup Brie cheese, chopped

1 white onion, diced

1 tsp. paprika

6 lettuce leaves

¼ cup butter, unsalted

1 tbsp. ghee

1 clove garlic, minced

Salt and pepper, to taste.

Directions

1. Mix the cream cheese and the butter in a food processor and transfer to a bowl. When finished mix in the Brie.

2. Add the onion and the garlic in a pan and cook for approximately 3 minutes over medium heat with the ghee. Let cool.

3. Once cooled, combine with the cheese and the butter mixture. Season with the spices and mix.

4. Refrigerate for a minimum of 30 minutes. Make 6 fat bombs out of the mixture.

5. Serve on lettuce leaves.

Nutrition

Calories 158 kcal | Protein: 3.3g | Fat: 16.2g | Carbs: 2g.

SAVORY FAT BOMBS

Prep time: 1 h
Cook time: 5 min
Servings: 06

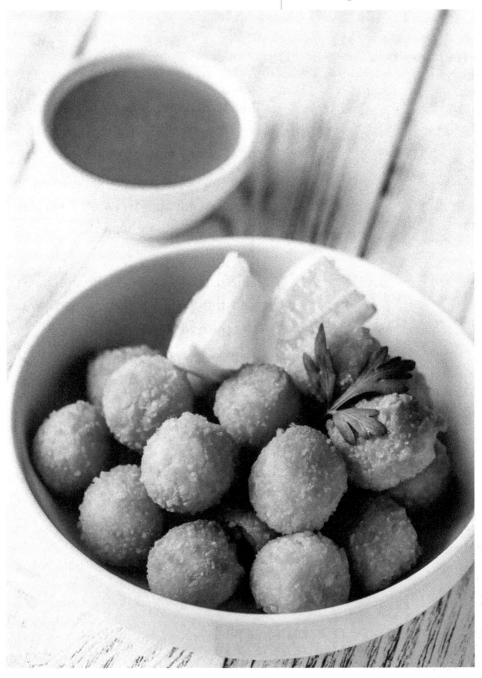

Ingredients

3.5 oz. cream cheese

¼ cup butter, cubed

2 large (2.1 oz.) slices of bacon

1 medium (0.5 oz) spring onion

1 clove garlic, crushed.

Directions

1. Add a cream cheese and butter to a bowl. Leave uncovered to soften at room temperature.

2. While that softens, set your bacon in a skillet on medium heat and cook until crisp. Allow it to cool then crumble into small pieces.

3. Add in your remaining ingredients to your cream cheese mixture and mix until fully combined.

4. Spoon small molds of your mixture onto a lined baking tray (about 2 tablespoons per mold). Then place to set in the freezer for about 30 minutes.

5. Set your Air Fryer to preheat to 350°F. Put in the Air Fryer basket with gap in between and cook for 5 minutes.

6. Cool to room temperature.

Nutrition

Calories 108 kcal | Protein: 2.1g | Fats: 11.7g | Carbs: 3.4g.

CHORIZO AND AVOCADO FAT BOMBS

Prep time: 45 min

Cook time: 8 min

Servings: 04

Ingredients

3.5 oz. Spanish Chorizo sausage, diced

¼ cup butter, unsalted

1 tbsp. lemon juice

Salt and cayenne pepper, to taste

2 large, hard-boiled eggs, diced

2 tbsp. mayonnaise

2 tbsp. chives, chopped

4 avocado halves, pitted.

Directions

1. Fry chorizo for 5 minutes in a hot pan. Set aside.

2. Combine all the ingredients in a mixing bowl and season with salt and cayenne pepper to taste. Mash together with a fork.

3. Refrigerate for approximately 30 minutes, and then fill each avocado half with ¼ of the mixture. Serve.

Nutrition

Calories 419 kcal | Protein: 11.4g | Fat: 38.9g | Carbs: 9.1g.

STUFFED ZUCCHINI

Prep time: 15 min
Cook time: 18 min
Servings: 08

Ingredients

4 medium zucchinis

1 cup red bell pepper

½ cup Kalamata olives

½ cup fresh tomatoes

1 tsp. garlic

1 tbsp. dried oregano

½ cup feta cheese, crumbled.

Directions

1. Preheat your oven to 350ºF. Grease a large baking sheet.

2. With a melon baller, spoon out the flesh of each zucchini half. Discard the flesh.

3. In a bowl, mix together the bell pepper, olives, tomatoes, garlic, oregano, salt, and black pepper.

4. Stuff each zucchini half with the veggie mixture evenly. Arrange zucchini halves onto the prepared baking sheet and bake for about 15 minutes.

5. Now, set the oven to broiler on high. Top each zucchini half with feta cheese and broil for about 3 minutes. Serve hot.

Nutrition

Calories 59 kcal | Fat: 3.2g | Carbs: 0.9g | Protein: 2.9g.

BROCCOLI WITH BELL PEPPERS

Prep time: 15 min

Cook time: 10 min

Servings: 06

Ingredients

2 tbsp. butter

2 garlic cloves, minced

1 large yellow onion, sliced

3 large red bell peppers

2 cups small broccoli florets

1 tbsp. low-sodium soy sauce

¼ cup homemade vegetable broth.

Directions

1. In a large wok, melt butter oil over medium heat and sauté the garlic for about 1 minute.
2. Add the vegetables and stir fry for about 5 minutes.
3. Stir in the broth and soy sauce and stir fry for about 4 minutes or until the desired doneness of the vegetables.
4. Stir in the black pepper and remove from the heat. Serve hot.

Nutrition

Calories 74 kcal | Fat: 4.1g | Carbs: 14g | Protein: 2.1g.

MUSHROOMS AND SPINACH

Prep time: 10 min

Cook time: 10 min

Servings: 04

Ingredients

10 oz. spinach leaves

14 oz. mushrooms

2 garlic cloves

½ cup fresh parsley

1 onion

4 tbsp. olive oil

2 tbsp. balsamic vinegar.

Directions

1. Heat a pan with the oil over medium-high heat, add the garlic and onion, stir, and cook for 4 minutes.

2. Add the mushrooms, stir, and cook for 3 minutes.

3. Add the spinach, stir, and cook for 3 minutes.

4. Add the vinegar, salt, and pepper, stir, and cook for 1 minute.

5. Add the parsley, stir, divide between plates, and serve.

Nutrition

Calories 200 kcal | Fat: 4g | Carbs: 7.6g | Protein: 13.5g.

BRUSSELS SPROUTS AND BACON

Ingredients

8 bacon strips, chopped

1-pound Brussels sprouts

A pinch of cumin

A pinch of red pepper, crushed

2 tbsp. extra virgin olive oil.

Directions

1. Toss Brussels sprouts with salt, pepper, cumin, red pepper, and oil to coat.

2. Spread the Brussels sprouts on a lined baking sheet, place in an oven at 375ºF, and bake for 30 minutes.

3. Heat a pan over medium heat, add the bacon pieces, and cook them until they become crispy.

4. Divide the baked Brussels sprouts on plates, top with bacon, and serve.

Nutrition

Calories 256 kcal | Fat 20g | Carbs: 7.6g | Protein: 32.2g.

INDIAN CAULIFLOWER RICE

Prep time: 5 min

Cook time: 20 min

Servings: 06

Ingredients

⅓ cup Ghee

2 garlic cloves, minced

½-inch Ginger, finely chopped

½ tsp ground turmeric

½ tsp. cumin seeds

1 tsp. coriander seeds

½ tsp. yellow mustard seeds

½ tsp. brown mustard seeds

26 oz. cauliflower processed into rice

2 tbsp. cilantro, chopped

Salt and black pepper, to taste

Directions

1. Into a large non-stick frying pan over medium-high heat sauté the ghee, garlic and ginger and until fragrant.

2. Add all of the spices and sauté for 3 to 5 minutes.

3. Gently mix in half of the cauliflower rice and sauté for 3 minutes. Then stir in the remaining cauliflower rice.

4. Season with salt and pepper to taste and cook for another 8-10 minutes, mixing continuously, until softened.

5. Remove from heat and add the chopped cilantro. Serve hot.

Nutrition

Calories 224 kcal | Fat: 12g | Carbs: 7g | Protein: 4g.

AVOCADO SAUCE

Ingredients

2 oz. pistachio nuts

1 tsp. salt

¼ cup lime juice

2 tbsp. garlic, minced

¼ cup water

⅔ cup olive oil

1 avocado

1 cup fresh parsley or cilantro.

Directions

1. Use a food processor or a blender to mix all of the ingredients together until they are smooth except the pistachio nuts and olive oil.

2. Add these at the end and mix well. If the mix is a bit thick add in a bit more oil or water.

Nutrition

Calories 490 kcal | Fat 50g | Carbs: 7.6g | Protein 5g.

BLUE CHEESE DRESSING

Prep time: 1 h

Cook time: 0 min

Servings: 01

Ingredients

2 tbsp. parsley, fresh

1 tsp. black pepper

1 tsp. salt

½ cup heavy whipping cream

½ cup mayonnaise

¾ cup greek yogurt

5 oz. blue cheese.

Directions

1. Break the blue cheese up into small chunks in a large bowl.

2. Stir in the heavy cream, mayonnaise, and yogurt.

3. Mix in the parsley, salt, and pepper and let the dressing sit for 1 hour, so the flavors mix well.

4. This dressing will be good in the refrigerator for three days.

Nutrition

Calories 477 kcal | Fat: 47g | Carbs: 12.5g | Protein: 10g.

SATAY SAUCE

Ingredients

1 can coconut cream

1 dry red pepper, seeds removed, chopped fine

1 clove garlic, minced

¼ cup gluten-free soy sauce

⅓ cup natural unsweetened peanut butter

Salt and pepper.

Directions

1. Place all ingredients in a small saucepan.

2. Bring the mixture to a boil.

3. Stir while heating to mix peanut butter with other ingredients as it melts.

4. After the mixture boils, turn down the heat to simmer on low heat for 5 to 10 minutes.

5. Remove from heat when the sauce is at the desired consistency.

6. Adjust seasoning to taste.

Nutrition

Calories 158 kcal | Fat: 13g | Carbs: 5g | Protein: 7g.

SALSA DRESSING

Prep time: 1 h
Cook time: 0 min
Servings: 01

Ingredients

1 tbsp. garlic, minced

1 tsp. chili powder

3 tbsp. apple cider vinegar

2 tbsp. mayonnaise

2 tbsp. sour cream

¼ cup olive oil

½ cup salsa.

Directions

1. Mix all of the ingredients to a large bowl.
2. Pour into a glass jar and let the dressing chill in the refrigerator for at least one hour.

Nutrition

Calories 200 kcal | Fat: 21g | Carbs: 3.2g | Protein: 1g.

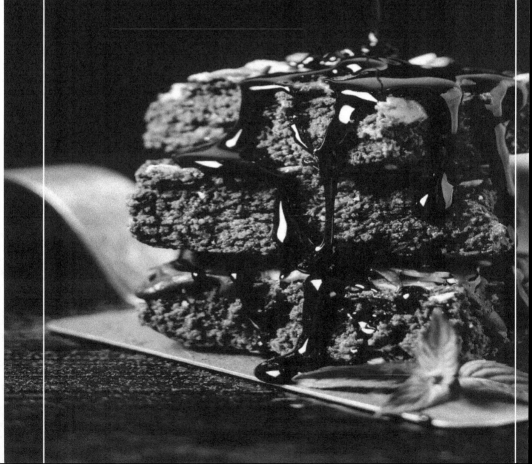

DESSERT RECIPES

EASY PEANUT BUTTER CUPS

Prep time: 10 min

Cook time: 1h 35min

Servings: 12

Ingredients

1/2 cup peanut butter

1/4 cup butter

3 oz. cacao butter, chopped

1/3 cup powdered swerve sweetener

1/2 tsp vanilla extract

4 oz. sugar-free dark chocolate.

Directions

1. Using low heat, melt the peanut butter, butter, and cacao butter in a saucepan. Stir them until thoroughly combined. Add the vanilla and sweetener until there are no more lumps.

2. Prepare muffin tin with parchment paper. Carefully place the mixture in the muffin cups. Refrigerate it until firm

3. Put chocolate in a bowl and set the bowl in boiling water. This is done to avoid direct contact with the heat. Stir the chocolate until completely melted.

4. Take the muffin out of the fridge and drizzle in the chocolate on top. Put it back again in the fridge to firm it up. This should take 15 minutes to finish.

5. Store and serve when needed.

Nutrition

Calories 200 kcal | Fat 19g | Carbs: 6g | Protein: 8g.

KETO MOCHA CHEESECAKE

Prep time: 10 min

Cook time: 0 min

Servings: 04

Ingredients

¾ cup heavy whipping cream

1 block of cream cheese (room temperature)

¼ cup unsweetened cocoa

¾ cup Swerve Confectioners sweetener

1 double shot of espresso.

Directions

1. Place the softened cream cheese in a bowl, and using a hand mixer, whip the cream cheese for 1 minute. Add espresso and continue mixing.

2. Add the sweetener, ¼ cup at a time and mix. Be sure to taste periodically, you may not need to use all the sweetener.

3. Add cocoa powder and mix until completely blended.

4. In a separate bowl, whip the cream until stiff peaks form.

5. Gently fold the whipped cream into the mocha mixture using a spatula. Place in individual serving dishes. Enjoy!

Nutrition

Calories 425 kcal | Protein: 6g | Fat: 33g | Carbs: 4.7g.

BLUEBERRY MUG CAKE

Prep time: 3 min

Cook time: 2 min

Servings: 02

Ingredients

2 tbsp. coconut flour

½ tsp. baking powder

25 grams fresh blueberries

1 large egg

2 tbsp. cream cheese

1 tbsp. butter

15 – 20 drips Liquid Stevia

¼ tsp. Himalayan Salt.

Directions

1. Add the butter and cream cheese to a mug and microwave for 20 seconds. Mix with a fork.

2. Add the baking powder, coconut flour and stevia and combine with a fork. Add the egg and combine.

3. Add the salt and fresh blueberries, and fold gently. Microwave for 90 seconds.

4. Eat right out of the mug or flip out onto a plate. For added flavor dust with powdered swerve.

Nutrition

Calories 345 kcal | Protein: 10g | Carbs: 8.7g | Fat: 29g.

LAVA CAKE

Prep time: 10 min

Cook time: 0 min

Servings: 01

Ingredients

2 oz. unsweetened dark chocolate

2 oz. unsalted butter

2 organic eggs

2 tbsp. powdered Erythritol

1 tbsp. almond flour.

Directions

1. Preheat the oven to 350°F.

2. Grease 2 ramekins. In a microwave-safe bowl, add the chocolate and butter and microwave on High for about 2 minutes, stirring after every 30 seconds. Remove from the microwave and stir until smooth.

3. Place the eggs in a bowl and with a wire whisk, beat well. Add the chocolate mixture, Erythritol, and almond flour, and mix until well combined.

4. Divide the mixture into the prepared ramekins evenly. Bake for approximately 9 minutes or until the top is set.

5. Remove the ramekins from oven and set aside for about 1–2 minutes. Carefully, invert the cakes onto the serving plates and dust with extra powdered Erythritol.

Nutrition

Calories 478 kcal | Fat: 44g | Carbs: 8.5g | Protein: 9.6g.

LOW CARB PECAN PIE

Prep time: 10 min
Cook time: 40 min
Servings: 12

Ingredients

For Crust

¼ cup butter

2 eggs

½ cup almond flour

¼ cup stevia

¼ tsp. salt

½ cup coconut flour

For Filling

¼ cup butter

2 eggs

½ cup sugar-free caramel syrup

¼ cup granular stevia

Directions

To Make a Crust

1. In a medium microwavable bowl, melt butter for 30 seconds.

2. Stir in eggs, almond flour, stevia and salt.

3. Add sifted coconut flour and mix well.

4. Knead the dough with your hands for 1 minute, then shape it into a ball.

5. Roll out between wax paper to about ⅛-inch think and turn it into 9-inch pie pan.

6. Preheat the oven to 325°F.

To Make a Filling

7. In a medium microwavable bowl, melt butter for 30 seconds.

8. Beat melted butter, eggs, caramel syrup, stevia, vanilla extract and salt until well combined.

2 tsp. vanilla extract

½ tsp. salt

1½ cup pecans, chopped

9. Stir in pecans.

10. Pour the mixture into the pie crust.

11. Bake for 35 to 40 minutes. The middle of the pie should not be set completely.

12. Let cool completely before serving.

Nutrition

Calories 250 kcal | Protein: 5.6g | Fat: 22g | Carbs: 4g.

LOW CARB BUTTER COOKIES

Prep time: 10 min

Cook time: 10 min

Servings: 06

Ingredients

1 cup almond flour

¼ cup Confectioners Swerve

3 tbsp. salted butter (room temperature)

½ tsp. vanilla extract.

Directions

1. Preheat oven to 350°F.

2. Prepare a baking sheet lined with parchment paper or a nonstick baking mat.

3. In a mixing bowl, combine all ingredients, stirring thoroughly until resembling a dough. (it will look crumbly while you stir, then will form into a cohesive dough).

4. Form 1-inch balls, placing them on the baking sheet. There should be about 12 balls, separated from each other by about 2 inches.

5. Flatten each dough ball using a fork, then rotate 90 degrees and flatten again, forming a crisscross pattern.

6. Bake at 350°F until the cookie are golden around the edges, 8-10 minutes depending on the thickness of the cookies.

7. Let cool completely before removing them from the baking

sheet, they cookies will be very soft when they first come out of the oven.

Nutrition

Calories 80 kcal | Protein: 2g | Fat: 8g | Carbs: 3.2g.

COCONUT & CHOCOLATE PUDDING

Prep time: 2 h 5 min

Cook time: 20 min

Servings: 06

Ingredients

2 egg yolks

14 oz. canned unsweetened coconut milk

1 tsp. vanilla extract

3 oz. sugar-free dark chocolate.

Directions

1. In a saucepan combine egg yolks and coconut milk and mix well. Place over medium low heat and let simmer while stirring for 10 minutes.

2. In a medium bowl add chocolate broken into small pieces and vanilla extract. Pour the coconut milk on top. Wait until the chocolate melts.

3. Whisk the batter and transfer into glasses.

4. Refrigerate for at least 2 hours before serving.

Nutrition

Calories 325 kcal | Protein: 5g| Carbs: 4.7g | Fat: 23g.

CPSIA information can be obtained
at www.ICGtesting.com
Printed in the USA
BVHW092301210621
610124BV00009B/1552

9 781802 993967